The ~~Worst~~ Best Year

The ~~Worst~~ Best Year

A Mother and Son's Obstacle Through Cancer

Natalie Khoury and Sebastian Khoury

The ~~Worst~~ Best Year - A Mother & Son's Obstacle Through Cancer

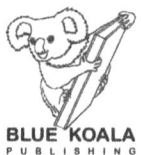

Text and Images Copyright © 2024
Natalie Khoury and Sebastian Khoury

All rights reserved. No part of this book may be reproduced, stored in a retrieval system, or transmitted in any form or by any means, electronic or mechanical, including photocopying, scanning, recording or otherwise, without permission in writing from the copyright owners.

ISBN 978-0-6486156-1-3

Authored and published by Natalie Khoury and Sebastian Khoury

Blue Koala Publishing
info@bluekoalapublishing.com

When something bad happens,
You have three choices.
You can either let it define you,
let it destroy you,
or you can let it strengthen you.

~ Dr Seuss

Special thanks to Michelle Musumeci, Karlana Kasarik, Anthony Harb, Olga Badawi, Angela Santopoli, Lanelle Eid, Jerome Khoury, Elijah Khoury and George Khoury for their guidance through the editing process and in getting this book to print.

A Note to the Reader

This book is a memoir. It reflects the authors' present recollections of experiences over time. Some names and characteristics have been changed, some events have been compressed, and some dialogue has been recreated. The authors' experiences may not be the same as yours and any claims made are how the authors remember them and may not be exactly how they unfolded.

The information, including but not limited to text, graphics, images, and other material in this book, is for information purposes only. No material in this book is intended to be a substitute for professional medical advice, diagnosis, or treatment. Always seek the advice of your physician or other qualified healthcare provider for answers to questions regarding a medical condition or treatment, and before undertaking a new healthcare regimen. Never disregard professional medical advice or delay seeking it because of something you have read in this book.

CHAPTERS

Introduction ~ *Natalie*	1
1) A Mother's Diagnosis ~ *Natalie*	6
2) Mum's First Obstacle ~ *Sebastian*	20
3) Let's Do Good ~ *Natalie*	23
4) The Itch ~ *Sebastian*	31
5) The Diagnosis ~ *Sebastian*	47
6) This Can't Be Happening Again ~ *Natalie*	63
7) Life Goes On, But The Tests Do Not Stop ~ *Natalie*	78
8) Are We Really Talking Fertility? ~ *Sebastian*	92
9) The First Day of Chemo ~ *Sebastian*	98
10) Cancer Didn't Make Us Sick, Chemo Did ~ *Natalie*	110
11) My Bones Are Dying ~ *Sebastian*	116
12) Chemo Leak ~ *Sebastian*	127
13) Cancer And Personal Life ~ *Sebastian*	144
14) The COVID Holiday ~ *Sebastian*	153
15) Cancer Changes More Than Looks ~ *Natalie*	172
16) Sickness And Transfusions ~ *Sebastian*	178
17) Cancer Kills More Than The Body ~ *Sebastian*	199
18) The Last Chemo ~ *Natalie*	208
19) Is The Journey Really Over? ~ *Sebastian*	216
20) So Many Wonderful Charities ~ *Natalie*	225
21) It's Never Over ~ *Sebastian*	232
22) Finding A New Normal ~ *Natalie*	244
Simply Put ~ *Sebastian*	251

Introduction

~ *Natalie* ~

Throughout my life, people always said, "You are so strong, Natalie!" When I had cancer, I heard this all the time, and then again when my son was diagnosed with cancer eight years later. Throughout these difficult times, I did not always feel strong. The irony is when someone says, "You are so strong," you feel you need to be. The truth is what appears on the surface does not always reflect what is happening underneath.

It is common for people to talk about their 'Cancer Journey'. My son Sebastian does not have an issue with this term. I detest it so much. A journey implies a choice, a path willingly embarked upon. Cancer doesn't offer that luxury. It is an unwelcome intruder, a path laid down before us and a path we never accepted. In 2013, I didn't choose cancer, and neither did Sebastian in 2022. Yet, despite the weight of this burden, we've faced it head-on, navigating the stormy waters it brings. This book isn't a narrative of a cancer journey; it's a testament to overcoming

The ~~Worst~~ Best Year

the obstacles that cancer forced upon me, my son, and my loved ones. These experiences have sculpted us into the individuals we are today and etched resilience into our souls, illuminating our strength.

After my diagnosis and during my treatment, I thought a lot about writing a book about my experiences. It was going to be called 'Through My Eyes - My Cancer Obstacle', and through the book I hoped to help those facing similar challenges. However, despite this longing to make a difference to others, the pathway to action seemed clouded in uncertainty. Translating my thoughts, emotions, and insights into tangible words that could resonate with others was daunting. Writing seemed a mountain too high to climb, overshadowed by doubts and insecurities. Amidst these doubts, though, I knew deep down that my story held the potential to inspire, comfort, and guide those navigating similar paths. So, despite my apprehension, I resolved to share my experiences in another way to offer a beacon of light to those travelling through darkness.

I chose to fundraise for cancer research and organised numerous morning teas for the Cancer Council. Giving back to the Cancer Council was important as they were my first port of call, helping me to digest and navigate what was to come, both medically and emotionally. Over the years, I raised a significant amount of money for cancer research and most importantly, I raised community awareness. The work I did as an Ambassador for the Cancer Council helped me find myself after cancer, as it gave me a sense of purpose behind my experience. Did I want cancer? No! Could I make the most of a challenging situation?

Natalie - Introduction

Yes, I could if I wanted to.

After my son Sebastian was diagnosed with cancer, I was filled with an overwhelming urge to write. This time, I envisioned a version of this book from both our perspectives, bringing us to the title 'Through Our Eyes - A Mother and Son's Cancer Obstacle', but that name was taken. We wanted a unique title, so we opted for 'The ~~Worst~~ Best Year', which sums up our experiences. As humans, we always look for reasons as to why things occur, and situations can be viewed in many ways, sometimes even as both bad and good. In my search for a reason, I was blaming God. My logical brain knew that God did not give this to us, but amid our challenges, I couldn't help but feel that way; I could not fathom why God would let this happen to our family, not once, but twice. Sebastian does not overthink things like I do. He believes things just happen. This thought process was a real blessing. Our favourite saying became "It is what it is".

However, over time I have come to realise that I did things in my life that I never would have if it wasn't for my cancer diagnosis. Sebastian has said similar things. Throughout this obstacle, my son and I have encountered challenges that tested us in many ways and reshaped our perspectives on life. Yet, intertwined with the hardships were moments of profound beauty, unwavering love, and unexpected blessings. We've formed connections, unearthed strengths we never knew we possessed, and embraced the power of community in ways we never could have anticipated.

Sebastian was undergoing treatment during the pandemic, which

The ~~Worst~~ Best Year

created numerous roadblocks for us. Yet, it was when I had COVID and was isolating in my room that I saw it as an opportunity to make the most of my time. I finally started writing the book I had been dreaming about for the past nine years, the book I wanted to write for many reasons: I want cancer patients to know that they will find purpose behind their obstacles, maybe not now, but one day; I want mothers going through treatment to see that they are going to become stronger on the other side; I want the partner watching their loved one going through treatment to understand what they may be experiencing and feeling; I want the parents watching their child battle cancer to know that they are stronger than they think.

Our story, of course, has involved many other people, several to whom I want to extend profound expressions of gratitude. Firstly, to my cousin, Michelle, thank you for the endless nights of work and discussion that brought our story to life. I want to thank my parents and in-laws who have been unwavering pillars of support throughout every twist and turn in my life. Their love, guidance, and presence have helped me weather storms and celebrate triumphs.

To my three beautiful boys—Jerome, Sebastian, and Elijah—you are the essence of my being. Your boundless love, laughter, and resilience have been my guiding light, infusing each moment with hope and purpose. You have given me strength when I faltered and inspired me to continue fighting no matter the odds. My love for you knows no bounds.

And to my beloved husband, George. Your unwavering devotion and steadfast love have been my anchor amid life's turbulent seas. When we

Natalie - Introduction

exchanged vows in 2001 you promised for better or worse, in sickness and health, to stand by my side through every trial and tribulation, and you have more than honoured that promise. Your unshakeable support, comforting presence, and selfless acts of kindness have carried me through moments of despair and uncertainty. You have been my voice when I could not speak, my rock when I felt adrift, and my greatest source of strength and solace. Without you, I cannot fathom where I would be and I thank you for being my constant companion, my confidant, and my greatest blessing.

Everyone's path on a road like this is different and people experiencing cancer will have their own story. This is our story. This is how we felt. Yet this is more than just a story; it's a testament to the unwavering spirit that can emerge from life's most testing challenges. Cancer may have disrupted our lives, but it has also illuminated the path to profound self-discovery and renewal. Throughout these pages, we aim to unravel the complexities of our obstacles and extend a hand of understanding to those who walk a similar path. We hope opening up about our obstacles can help somebody going through a difficult time.

Chapter 1

A Mother's Diagnosis

~ Natalie ~

November 12th, 2013 marked a pivotal moment that forever altered my life. It wasn't a change full of negativity but rather a transformation that unfolded unexpectedly, in turn reshaping the very fabric of my existence. Prior to this date, I revelled in the joys of life, basking in the warmth of motherhood as I raised three vibrant boys with the help of my devoted husband. Our recent move into a new home symbolised the dawn of a fresh chapter brimming with hopes and dreams for our young family. Little did I know that just beyond the horizon lay an unforeseen twist of fate that would challenge me and my family in ways I never imagined.

It all started with me feeling tired and a persistent itch on my scalp. As a mother of three, I initially dismissed the tiredness as normal. I thought the itch was due to a sensitive scalp, but as it continued, I became convinced that I had insects living on my scalp, leading me to suspect the presence of head lice. The intensity of the itch was so extraordinary that I often asked George for help, urging him to inspect my hair for any signs of an infestation. However, this itch was the beginning of a much larger revelation.

That fateful Saturday morning of November 2nd, 2013, I awoke to a sharp pain in my neck; a sensation that in no way made me think of cancer, and was unrelated to the cancer that I would soon discover I had. As I applied Voltaren cream to alleviate the discomfort, an impulse made me massage the excess cream into the area near my collarbone. There, my fingers encountered a lump beneath the surface, similar in size to a Kalamata olive.

Instinctively, I asked George to inspect the lump, to provide a sense of reassurance amid my uncertainty. He dismissed my concerns with light-hearted banter, laughing it off as hypochondria. With a laugh, I warned him that if I died, he would be sorry that he didn't tell me to get the lump checked out. To this day, we still laugh about those comments as my situation's outcome allows us to do so.

Amid the chaos of organising my son Sebastian's 7th birthday celebration, I knew the right thing to do was to get the lump checked out as soon as possible. As a newcomer to the area, I found myself unexpectedly navigating the parking lot of a medical clinic unfamiliar to me. The receptionist informed me that there weren't any doctors available at that moment and suggested I return later in the day to see Dr Brenda at 1.00 pm.

Dr Brenda was professional and thorough but that did little to alleviate my concerns. During her investigation she felt the lump around my neck as well as inspecting my armpits and groin area. Upon concluding the examination, she gave me a slip requesting blood work and an ultrasound with a fine needle biopsy. My worries began to set in at this point and as fate would have it, the timing of my visit coincided with the eve of the Melbourne Cup. If you live in Australia, you know that the Melbourne Cup is 'the race that stops the nation' and with the public holiday long weekend, I wasn't able to get a biopsy appointment until Friday. I had a follow-up appointment with Dr Brenda on Thursday the week after to get the results. Unexpectedly on Monday afternoon, I received a phone call from the clinic informing me that a different doctor would see me on Tuesday, as my results were in and that it could not wait until Thursday. I instantly felt a knot in my stomach. Deep down I knew with a phone call like that the news awaiting me would not be favourable. Yet, despite this intuition, I was in denial and refusing to entertain the possibility of bad news.

The appointment was in the afternoon so I told George I would meet him there as he insisted on coming with me. George was caught in traffic and the doctor told me to go straight in as soon as I arrived at the clinic. He wasted no time saying, "I have booked an appointment for you tonight with your regular haematologist, Dr Steve. He will have all your results." I was feeling very confused as Dr Steve had been treating me for low platelets for some time. My platelet issue was unrelated to cancer but he was also an oncologist, so why would I be going there? "Why am I going to see Dr Steve? Is there a problem with my platelets?" I asked.

To which he replied, "No, you have Hodgkin lymphoma". Just like that! Seriously, just like that! I think he thought I knew my diagnosis. I said, "HODGKIN'S!!!! Is that cancer?" He replied, "Yes," and pushed a box of tissues towards me. Only three times in my life have I had an out-of-body experience. This was the first. The second was the day my dad passed away, and the third was the moment I was told my son Sebastian had cancer. It's like everyone around you is talking but all you hear is white noise. The words people say are muffled and the white noise is deafening. I couldn't shake the feeling that I was living in a scene from a movie where the main character grapples with the reality of impending doom. I found myself living out a narrative in real-time, the weight of that impending doom bearing upon me with an intensity like no other. I know I sound dramatic but that's exactly how I felt. You only know this feeling if you have experienced it. I walked out of the clinic completely numb. Did this doctor just say I have cancer? What the f**k? I can't have cancer! He must be wrong!

I rang George from the car park and told him I was headed to Dr Steve's office because I have cancer, an expression I uttered with no emotion or feeling. I cannot remember his exact words, but he asked me to go home and wait for him there. From the moment I left the GP's office until I arrived at Dr Steve's office was all a blur. I was pacing like a mad woman up and down the hallway at home waiting for him. I had so many thoughts running through my head. I kept thinking: *I cannot have cancer. I cannot have cancer. The doctor must have it wrong. I do*

The ~~Worst~~ Best Year

not feel sick. How can I have cancer?

When George walked through the door, I yelled at him for being late and said we had to go. Dr Steve wasn't waiting for us. He was just going to fit us in when we arrived, but I was overcome with all these emotions and did not know how to express my feelings. We often take out our frustrations on those closest to us and in that moment in time, I needed to hear what Dr Steve thought of the situation. Every part of me was hoping that the GP was wrong, and Dr Steve was going to tell me, "Do not worry, you are going to be fine". The drive to the clinic passed in a complete haze as the familiar landmarks and bustling streets reduced to a blur of indistinct shapes and colours. What I do remember is feeling fear. I knew with a chilling certainty that my life would never be the same again. I knew that an invisible line had been crossed, a point of no return marking the onset of a new chapter fraught with uncertainty and upheaval.

The wait to see Dr Steve was long. When we were finally called in, he was very reassuring. He said until we do the PET scan and remove the growth, we cannot be 100% sure of what we are dealing with, but if it is Hodgkin lymphoma, the prognosis is good. What came next was a rollercoaster. I had to get a bone marrow test to make sure that the cancer had not spread to my bones. That in itself was a challenging experience, and I was petrified about this as I had heard it was very painful. Painful it was, but it was over quickly enough. Then came the surgery to remove the cancerous lymph node, a PET scan, blood tests, and appointment after appointment.

Natalie - A Mother's Diagnosis

It was the waiting that drove me crazy. The wait time felt so long but looking back, I realise the process took about two weeks, and then I had my answer. In hindsight, it was not long at all. I was diagnosed with stage 1A nodular sclerosis, classical Hodgkin lymphoma. Dr Steve expressed that "because I was a hypochondriac" and caught it early, the treatment plan would be six rounds (three cycles) of a chemotherapy combination called ABVD (Doxorubicin, Bleomycin, Vinblastine, Dacarbazine) and 15 days of radiation. He went on to explain that this type of cancer usually gets diagnosed in more advanced stages, so I was lucky I found the lump on my neck. Now I had an answer to the itchy scalp, as this was one of the symptoms of the disease that a lot of lymphoma patients complain about.

The surgery removed the whole cancer and this was good news. However, I still had to go through the entire treatment plan, which would prove to be intense. The doctor explained: "Imagine your cancer being a weed; you pull it out, but if you do not apply the weed kill, it can come back." It made sense, but this was going to be tough. I first asked Dr Steve, "Am I going to lose my hair?" How vain is that? Seriously, am I going to lose my hair? Looking back, who gives a shit? Losing my hair was tough but it was the least of my problems. The second thing I asked him was, "Am I going to survive?" He informed me that I would lose my hair, but the prognosis was good. Of course, doctors never promise anything. Dr Steve was honest and straightforward, explaining that the next few months would be inconvenient. I remember the word 'inconvenient' clearly and thought it was a funny way to describe the process. I personally would have added the word 'shit' before the word 'inconvenient.' That pretty much summed up the road ahead.

At this stage, I was almost 38 years old, and my boys were only nine, seven, and two. I never thought that I would receive a cancer diagnosis. Nobody ever thinks they're going to be diagnosed with cancer. How was I going to be a mother and undergo chemotherapy and radiation? My youngest was still in nappies and it felt impossible. When I first found out, I would cry in the shower so no one would hear me. I never wanted to cry in front of the boys. That would have caused them to be scared and as a result, they would have worried about me. I needed them to see how strong I was even though my world was falling apart.

We had to be honest with them, as they knew something was happening. We spent an extended amount of time at the hospital and had countless doctor appointments so we couldn't possibly hide what was happening. Telling my boys was so hard. Once we had all the facts, we explained to them what was happening to me in the simplest of terms. Jerome asked if it was stage four and whether that meant I would die. I was taken aback by that question and tried not to react when he asked, but I quickly assured him that I wouldn't die and that I would be receiving more treatment. I explained that this treatment would make me sick, and I would lose my hair, but in the end, the treatment would ensure that the cancer did not come back. They seemed okay after we shared the news with them. We spoke positively and told them to ask us any questions that they may have and I think that really helped in making them feel at ease. The boys showed resilience throughout my

Natalie - A Mother's Diagnosis

entire treatment.

My first chemotherapy session was on December 12th, a couple of weeks before Christmas. How unfair was that? I attended the school Christmas Carols with a vomit bag in my handbag as I was doing my best to keep that Christmas normal. That night I put a brave smile on my face and sang Christmas carols but I felt so nauseous. It took a while to get the anti-nausea medication right, yet I had to soldier on for my boys. Christmas was the happiest time of the year, and my illness was not going to get in the way of the joy and happiness that Christmas time brings!

I remember the exact moment they hooked me up to chemotherapy for the first time. I asked George to grab me a coffee and as soon as he left, they started to flush the first bag through my veins. I broke down and started to cry; this was now real. I had been bottling up all the fear of the day but couldn't any longer. So many times before this, from the moment I was diagnosed, I had cried into my pillow or in the shower, but this was now my reality. I had f**ing cancer. How was this possible? I lived a mostly healthy life, I was a good person, but as we have learnt, cancer does not discriminate. The chemotherapy nurse was a beautiful Irish woman. She comforted me while I let it all out. I felt better after that cry and it was then that I decided I had to toughen up and fight this horrible disease. This was my reality; I could sit and cry and ask, "Why me?" but it wouldn't help. As I sat there, I contemplated what if it had been one of my children going through this and knew that was something I could not accept. At that point I thanked God for giving this disease to me and sparing my boys. I had to believe that if someone in my family was going to get this horrible disease, then I was glad it was me. It was this thought at that very moment that made this entire experience bearable.

Chemotherapy took about four to five hours and was administered once a fortnight. It was delayed a couple of times due to my low white blood cell count and particularly my neutrophils, a type of white blood cell that is part of the immune system and helps the body fight infection. I was so disappointed the first time it was delayed as I just wanted the nightmare to end. When I was first told it was six rounds of chemotherapy, I asked how many months it would take. I wanted a time frame, but my doctor would not give me one and informed me that with this kind of treatment there would be delays due to blood count and other issues. He said if a time frame was put on it, I would only get disappointed whenever it was delayed. Even without the time frame for the treatment, I was extremely disappointed when it was delayed. "You work by cycles," Dr Steve told me. Every two treatments was one cycle and once a cycle starts, it generally doesn't stop.

George and Mum took it in turns to come with me. My Aunty Mary came in once to give them a break. I know how hard that would have been for her as this was the place she used to bring her late husband, Uncle George, to have his chemotherapy treatment. Losing him to cancer was devastating and this would have brought back a lot of sad memories for her. I had watched Uncle George suffer and this scared me a lot. I knew that Hodgkin had a better prognosis than some of the other types of cancers, but it was still cancer. Aunty Mary being by my side meant a lot to me and it was nice having someone there, but I hated seeing the sadness in everyone's eyes while they sat with me. Most of the time I slept, but it was just comforting to know someone was always with me. I had to stay in the hospital for roughly five hours for treatment and the nurses would offer me scones with butter and jam and make me a warm cup of tea. Everything I ate repeated on me and tasted metallic. By round four I refused to eat or drink anything and was happy to sleep through it all. After the treatment finished, when I saw a scone, it would take me back to that dreaded treatment room and it took me many years before I started eating them again.

I was receiving chemotherapy through a cannula in my hand. The medical staff always inserted it in my left hand as I was right-handed. I needed to be extremely careful not to dislodge it because if the chemo leaked on my skin, it would have dire effects. Going to the bathroom was not easy but there was no way to avoid it as you are pumped with so much fluid you just have to go. The first time I went to the bathroom after I received the chemotherapy my urine was blood red. They call it 'the red devil' (Doxorubicin). Luckily, they warned me before I went to the bathroom or I would have had a heart attack!

I didn't start losing my hair straight away but when it began to fall out, it was tough. I had imagined it coming out in chunks as soon as I started treatment, but that was not the case. Soon after round one, I began to feel a pinching sensation on my scalp and that's when my hair began to gradually shed. I would wake up and find hair on my pillow. I used to get so annoyed with the little strands that came out at the beginning. One afternoon, we were at a park with my cousin Carol from Sydney whose husband Peter is a hairdresser. He saw how I was pulling the strands out and picking them off my clothes. "Let's go find a pair of scissors and cut your hair short so it will be less annoying," he suggested. For many years prior, I would say to Carol, "I should get Peter to cut my hair short" but I never dared to do this. Losing my hair forced me to cut it and surprisingly, I really liked the way it looked. My hair had not been that short since I was a little child.

I remember walking into Dr Steve's office just before my third round of treatment and he said, "Wow! You Lebanese women have good genes; your hair is hanging in there!" But between rounds three and four of chemotherapy, I started to get patchy spots on my scalp. My body hair had already completely fallen out, something I did not mind at all. By this stage I had started to put on weight as I was on steroids as part of the chemotherapy treatment and Filgrastim injections to boost my blood count as it was always low. So, my prognosis was I was going bald and putting on weight. This was a big struggle because I put on nine kilograms in five months. I would sometimes get a glimpse of myself in the mirror and cry. I did not look like me anymore and I had very few photos taken during that period. As a woman, I found grappling with the vanity aspect quite challenging. Looking back now, I realise I let that side of things consume me but at the time that's how I felt.

George noticed that I was avoiding the mirror. One day, he told me he was going to the shops—and returned with a shaved head. When he walked in I gasped and asked, "What have you done?" "It's only hair," he replied. I can tell you, I fell in love with him all over again that day. It was a small gesture that meant so much. Our boys wanted to join in too, so off they all went to the barber. When they returned, we were a family with shaved heads. As a human race we can be so superficial and vain with our looks, and yet I have a family photo of us with shaved heads, and there are no filters. Elijah is in his nappy and we are all smiling. In my eyes, when looking at this photo we are the most beautiful family. It epitomises pure love and joy as you can see our love for each other and our joy for life. We honestly forget the simple things in life, things such as our hair colour or body shape, the size of our nose or the wrinkles on our face are not important. Nothing is important except for our health and the health of our family.

I wish I had kept a diary of my thoughts and my emotions at the time. It would have been nice to reflect and see how I felt on particular days. I kept a symptom diary just to keep track of how I was feeling physically after each treatment, but I felt shit most of the time to be honest. From day one to four of each treatment the nausea was horrible. On the day of the last treatment, I had to take Diazepam on the way to the hospital to calm my nerves as the anticipation of the nausea that resulted from each treatment was causing anxiety on my way to chemotherapy. I was always fatigued and constantly suffered from heartburn. My chemotherapy treatment was administered over the summer and I recall one night the heartburn was so extreme that I took my top off and lay on my stomach on the cold floor tiles to get some relief. I suffered from agonising constipation and my teeth became super sensitive to everything. Even my nails turned purple, but I soldiered on and by March, I had finished my chemotherapy treatment.

I had a few weeks off in between before the commencement of my radiation treatment. Now that was an experience! The hospital staff moulded a mask to my face that covered my head and shoulders. The mask went over my head and shoulders and locked onto the table while I underwent the radiation. I was locked in so tight it made me realise how precise and accurate the radiation beams needed to be. It's quite scary when I think about it. A bell was placed in my hand, and I was instructed that if I needed anything, to ring it and the treatment would be stopped. The first time I underwent the process, I struggled and almost rang it, but instead I recited about ten Hail Mary and ten Our Father prayers, and it was over. When the mask was unclipped, I had indentations on my face for about an hour after each treatment. That is how tight the mask was. This treatment happened Monday to Friday for three weeks. I found the radiation process much easier once I got used to being locked into the mask. Thankfully, I did not feel sick during this process so I could drive myself to and from the hospital. I was only fatigued from the radiation and I handled it a lot better than chemotherapy.

May 1st, 2014 marked a pivotal day in my life as I was completely finished with my treatment. I had a post-treatment scan that showed that I was cancer-free and I was now cleared of this horrible disease. I said, "Thank you God, We are done". Our family had endured its stint with cancer, and it was all over. At that moment, life was good again! I was going to go out into the world and do good things—things that would make a positive impact, however small, on the lives of others!

Chapter 2

Mum's First Obstacle

~ *Sebastian* ~

When my mother was diagnosed with Hodgkin lymphoma, I was only a young child. I have few memories of that time; however, I do remember feeling that everything was a bit different and life was changing for my family.

I remember when my mother and father first told me about the cancer diagnosis. My brother Jerome and I were called into our parents' room. Walking through the door, everything felt a little uneasy, like my insides were being played with and rearranged. You could tell something had happened and we weren't sure if we were in trouble. I started reflecting on everything I had done recently to make sure I wasn't about to get told off, but nothing came to mind. My parents were sitting down, anxiously waiting for us to join them. They tried to explain cancer to us, describing what it was and what it meant. I can't remember just how much I knew about cancer at the time, although

Sebastian - Mum's First Obstacle

what I do remember is that I really didn't connect with what they were saying. I had no experience with cancer at the time and knew nothing about it, so when they told my brother and me about Mum's diagnosis, I didn't think it was that big of a deal. However, even to young me, it was apparent that they were doing their best to conceal their inner angst and reassure us that everything was fine. While my recollection from this period is limited at best, their emotions and facial expressions have still stuck with me. They seemed overly worried about what was happening, my dad constantly pausing whilst speaking, emphasising just how big of a deal this was, but I still couldn't fully appreciate what was happening and why it was such a big deal.

After Mum's diagnosis, there were many changes. My mother, once a bright and cheerful person, was grappling with one of the most traumatic and troublesome journeys a person can travel, and as I was only seven I was ignorant of the magnitude of the situation. Despite understanding cancer on a basic level, I didn't realise what this demanded of a person or the people supporting them. Nevertheless, the emotions of my parents stood out. Whenever someone is going through something that you don't understand, rather than trying to learn everything there is to know about the subject, it's best to know what they are feeling and offer support to help them feel better in a way that makes sense for you. For me, maybe this meant getting my mum a glass of water when she was stuck on the couch and unable to move. This was a favour repaid many times over with hefty interest when I was the sick person stuck on the couch.

The ~~Worst~~ Best Year

One way our family thought about doing good was through solidarity. One of the changes that my mum was dealing with at the time was having to live with a shaved head. Transitioning from long, curly hair to short hair and then to no hair was really going to be a challenge for her. So our immediate family chose to step in and show support. My dad, older brother, younger brother, and I all decided to get buzz cuts. The thought of standing together was important for my mum, who felt weak at the time. After the cut, we took a family photo to capture the experience.

Looking back on that photo I see that our family seemed happy on the surface. Looking around and seeing everyone's shaved heads, I had the impression that we were one team, and our buzz-cuts were our uniform. *It was the Khoury identity, and I would later discover that the next time we had to play a game when I was diagnosed with cancer, we would all show up together in full uniform. Upon my diagnosis, all the men in my family chose to do the same for me. From my immediate family to my uncles, they all proved that even though the chemo entered my veins, its pain was shared by a legion of Khourys.* I guess if you ever see a bunch of my family walking around with shaved heads it's safe to assume that one of them has cancer.

Chapter 3

Let's Do Good

~ *Natalie* ~

When my cancer treatment ended, I felt an overwhelming sense of gratitude and the promise of renewal and healing. You imagine this moment to be perfect and joyous. You imagine you receive your results and the doctor congratulates you. You did it. You beat the beast! You embrace your support person, arrive home, tell everyone and they are completely overjoyed.

But it is not like that. When I received my results, I was so relieved that it was over, but I knew deep down within my heart that it was only just the beginning of my cancer obstacle. I felt this way because my oncologist had already booked me in for my next scans and blood tests, which would take place three months later. This was going to be a regular occurrence for the next five years at least. That night, I remember asking George: "What if they didn't get it all? I cannot go through that experience again." Despite the all-clear from the doctors,

The ~~Worst~~ Best Year

I had a deep fear of the cancer returning. Every single night I would feel for lumps. If I had a knot in my neck I would panic and think it had returned. This continued for a long time, but that overwhelming sense of fear eased as time passed. Just when I began to feel somewhat normal again, another routine scan would be due to take place, and my anxiety would set in. From the moment I completed the routine scan to the time I received the results, I would feel nauseous and sleep was non-existent. Again, as time passed—and I mean a lot of time—my anxiety improved. I never did receive any counselling despite the advice offered by others; I just soldiered on!

I found that giving back to the community gave my cancer a purpose. I completed radiation on May 1st 2014. In June, I hosted a 'Biggest Morning Tea' for the Cancer Council fundraising and extended an open invitation to anyone who wanted to attend. I had about 50 people join in celebrating my recovery with the aim of helping others, and I raised over $3,000 just by hosting this humble gathering in my dining room. I purchased an apron from the Cancer Council, which my guests signed with messages of support and congratulations. To this day, that apron means more than just a piece of fabric; it serves as a reminder of resilience, love, and the bonds that unite us as friends and family. It was such a rewarding afternoon, and I was buzzing at its completion. My heart was so whole, and I felt happy. I was proud to have raised so much money for such a fantastic cause. I sent an email to the Cancer Council with photos of our morning. This started a chain of events, and I became an Ambassador for the Cancer Council, telling my story to promote awareness and raise money through fundraising events.

My work as an Ambassador went on for the next three years, and I was able to experience moments that I had never imagined. Each year, I hosted a Biggest Morning Tea that was even bigger than the last, and I featured in online commercials and articles. I was raising awareness about being in tune with your body and not ignoring things that do not appear to be right. Raising funds was also helping to heal me from the post-traumatic stress that was lingering below the surface, which no one was aware of. It is not uncommon for cancer survivors to end up with post-traumatic stress, induced by the fear of cancer returning. The anger of what you go through. The frustration of your body never being the same, and let's not forget the survival guilt. I remember a beautiful man from our local milk bar who passed away soon after I finished treatment. When I went to give my condolences to his wife, I found out that he had died from cancer. I actually felt guilty. Of course I was happy that I had beaten this disease, but in that moment I realised that not everyone was as lucky as I was. This young family had just lost their father. This woman, who was of a similar age to me, had just lost her life partner. This man used to always enquire about my health, ask how I was feeling and was always so happy to know that things were going well. This gave me an even bigger drive to keep promoting the cause.

The following year, my living room was not big enough for our Biggest Morning Tea, so my children's primary school offered to host the event in the school hall. There I raised over $5,000. At these events we had guest speakers that told their stories. My story was in no way

The ~~Worst~~ Best Year

unique, and many people in our community had experienced their own struggles. We had children who spoke about watching their parents experience cancer and we had mothers from the school who shared their stories. Unfortunately, not all the stories had happy endings. A year later, the school offered use of the hall again and this time my husband George was the guest speaker. He told a story of a husband watching his wife go through cancer. He didn't include names; he shared about the impact this cancer diagnosis had on the people in the story. It was chilling, beautiful and moving, and at one point, I forgot it was about us.

George's story moved the parish priest so much that he informed us he would do a special collection at Mass on the weekend. That weekend, the priest was celebrating 25 years of priesthood and as it was a milestone occasion, many people were going to attend. With the special church collection and the money raised from the day of the event, we raised well over $9,000. The Biggest Morning Tea events I hosted continued over the years and with the Ambassadorial work that I undertook, I went from strength to strength. I was able to find myself again after cancer. Cancer patients would approach me saying that I had inspired them throughout their own treatment. My heart was overwhelmed with gratitude that I had the opportunity to make a difference in the lives of others who were struggling. Who would have thought that five years earlier I would be doing this kind of work? It is funny how life takes us down roads we never dreamed we would travel.

I spoke at many Morning Tea events aimed at raising funds and awareness. One of the first public speeches I gave was to a group of people I did not know. It was an event put on by the Cancer Council to launch Australia's Biggest Morning Tea fundraising month. My mother and my dear friend Mercy came along for moral support, and I was extremely grateful to share this experience with these two beautiful ladies who were by my side throughout this whole ordeal. I was a little nervous to speak but excited to help raise funds for this wonderful organisation. As I was speaking, I looked around the room and I saw some smiles as well as tears. They even laughed at some of my jokes! People nodded in understanding, and in that moment, I knew I had connected with many people with similar experiences. I had turned a bad situation into a good one and I was building awareness and raising funds at the same time. This was a positive in the fight against cancer.

Celebrity chef Darren Purchese was in the room that day with his partner Cath. I was a little bit of a fan as I had seen him on TV and loved the desserts he made. I have always enjoyed baking, and it's something that I'm good at—so I have been told. I was hoping at some point I could make my way over to introduce myself. When my speech was finished, I saw him walking towards me with Cath. Although I was extremely nervous, I managed to pull off looking calm and collected. They thanked me for sharing my story and asked if I would come to speak at their Morning Tea fundraiser at the Langham Hotel in two weeks. Ummm, Yeah! I didn't even stop to think. My mother quickly jumped in and asked, "Does mum get to come along too?" Mum is not backwards in coming forwards. "Of course!" Cath graciously replied, and I was happy to have my support queen accompany me.

The ~~Worst~~ Best Year

My mother always treated me like a princess and she will always be my queen. I may have been in my late thirties when I was diagnosed, but both my father and mother were always by my side like I was still that little girl who used to live with them. I will never forget my father's hugs, telling me I would be fine. He was so strong throughout my entire treatment. Anyone who knew my father knew he always wore his heart on his sleeve. He was a true Piscean and never hid his emotions. He loved with all his heart. I actually don't think he loved anyone or anything more than he loved me. (Sorry Mum!) When he hugged me and told me I would be fine, I felt that to be true.

The night before Darren and Cath's Morning Tea, I did not sleep! I was so nervous and went over my speech countless times. When we arrived, we walked into a beautifully presented room decorated elegantly in blue, white and yellow. Large round white tables filled the space, and the desserts were nothing short of divine! Darren was the superstar of dessert making. He baked for celebrities, and at that time he owned a beautiful shop in South Yarra called *Burch and Purchese*. The event's ambience was one of grace and elegance, fitting for the people being honoured. My mother and I were at the front table with the staff from the Cancer Council. The waiters went around offering champagne. I declined as it was still early morning and I had not eaten yet. Anyone who knows me knows I am a lightweight when it comes to drinking alcohol, but my mother was very happy to accept a glass. The MC began her introductions, and I was so nervous that I downed Mum's glass of champagne before I went up to the podium! Luckily, I had the podium to lean on to hide my shaking hands. I gave my speech and to be honest, I cannot remember the details of how it unfolded; that was how nervous I was! I was so relieved when it was over, but extremely grateful to have been given the opportunity to be involved in such a wonderful experience.

Later that year, George and I were invited to the Emerald and Ivy Ball in Sydney. This was a ball that Ronan Keating put on in honour of his mother, who passed away from breast cancer. It was absolutely a night to remember. We were rubbing shoulders with celebrities like Ronan and Storm Keating, Kylie Gillies, Chris Isaac, Darren Purchese and James Blunt, just to name a few. The room was decked out in emerald and ivy decorations, beautiful candelabras, and let's not forget Darren Purchese's edible centrepieces. That night I met a young lady, Nikki. This beautiful girl was diagnosed with leukaemia as a child and after having a reaction to the chemotherapy, her organs began to shut down. Her treatment was full of uncertainty that moved between hope and despair. She was now a gorgeous young lady and role model who spoke in a room full of celebrities, and she was the biggest superstar in the room. She shared her story, explaining that her experience as a patient undergoing treatment for leukaemia had inspired her to become a chemotherapy nurse. I was in awe of her and what she had overcome. This gave me great strength knowing that if a young child could make good out of this horrible disease, I was going to continue to find my strength to do the same. I thought of this girl's mother and the strength that this woman must have had to witness her daughter fight for her

The ~~Worst~~ Best Year

life! At the time, I was thinking I would never be able to watch my child go through what they went through. I kept thanking God for giving me cancer instead of one of my boys, as a child should never have to go through such an experience and miss out on any part of their childhood. However, we do not know what the future holds, and we do not know how strong we are until we are placed in such a situation.

Chapter 4

The Itch

~ Sebastian ~

Burning, fire, agony—my skin was ignited by an immune response and I was itching up a storm. It felt as though I was going to tear a hole through my skin. "Are you okay, Sebastian?" asked my schoolteacher. How could I be okay when I was itching like there was no tomorrow? Unfortunately, this was not a once-off incident. I had been itching like this on and off for a little while now and all I wanted was answers.

It was in and out of the doctor's office for several months. I had been experiencing chest pains only a week after my first dose of the Pfizer COVID-19 vaccine. This was known to have the side effect of myocarditis in a select few cases. Such circumstances prompted my first visit to see the local GP. The waiting room there always annoyed me; the walls, carpet, chairs, and people were so plain and dull. The only places with splashes of colour were the children's section and the TV fixed to the ABC Kids channel. You were constantly surrounded by sick, elderly people coughing and sneezing with no reprieve, and all you wanted was your name to be called so you could see the doctor. Whenever I heard someone walking down the corridor, I would jump up a little and sit nice and straight like the school principal had just entered the classroom, desperately hoping that my name would be called. Most of the time, I wouldn't be so lucky. After a little while, usually no less than half an hour of waiting, we would hear footsteps coming down the hallway one last time followed by the magic words, "Sebastian, just down the hall and take your fourth left". The wait was finally over.

The doctor I was seeing was new to me. We had recently been in between GPs, and given the potential urgency of my medical condition at the time, my mum chose to book the earliest available appointment rather than shop around for a doctor. My doctor noted that I had a very minor level of inflammation in the blood and performed some other tests to ensure that I was not in any imminent danger. He didn't seem too concerned with anything going on then and so there wasn't much to be noted. I ended up getting a scan that pointed to the chest pain originating from a recent injury. To be fair, it probably was.

***

Here we go again. This time my chest was not the culprit as I was pinched by a thousand itches simultaneously around my upper body. Before long, my fingers were tearing holes down to my legs, as if my limbs were attached to a remote control and a two-year-old toddler was button mashing the controller. I had to take my shirt off to see what damage the itching had done. To my surprise, my abdominal muscles were lined in a road of hives and red marks, some from my own itching, while some had ostensibly appeared on their own. I went downstairs, wearing no shirt with hesitancy as I sought my parent's help.

"Mum! Dad! I have these red spots everywhere and I don't know why."

"Don't worry Sebastian, your father gets those all the time after he has some garlic the night before. Take a Telfast (an antihistamine) and you will be fine." Sure enough, I took the Telfast and the itching soon dissipated.

I found myself getting ready for bed one evening. The warmth of the shower was always something I looked forward to at the end of my day. I often spent long, unnecessary periods in there at peace. This particular night, I was in the shower, turning up the heat and resting my head against the wall. The splashing on my neck gave me relief akin to scratching an itch. Having stood under the warm water for ten minutes, I'd thought it best to start lathering myself in body soap since I had only managed to apply shampoo so far. As I bent down to get some soap, my head strongly connected with the shower door handle. "Bang!" The thumping sound from the door caught me off guard, especially since everything was so calm only moments prior. I made contact with the handle in such a way that it jolted straight back causing immense shock. Aside from the initial startle, I had a minor headache.

It was around 10.00 pm, which was usually about the time I was getting ready for bed, not really in the mood to be treating a head injury, but my mother insisted that I stay awake for 45 minutes due to the knock to my head. I figured it wouldn't hurt too much, so I spent the next little while in our upstairs TV room, not watching TV but staring at a blank wall, ice pack on my head, until my mother was satisfied that it was safe to go to sleep.

Not surprisingly, I awoke the next morning to a round, red lump protruding from my upper forehead, prompting another visit to the doctor for a potential concussion. Again, I was forced to sit in the unpleasant waiting room, disappointed time after time as everyone else was called in. The doctor again noted very minor levels of inflammation in my blood, but thankfully, no signs of concussion. Another positive sign was that the already minor inflammation had begun to subside. Since I had recently had low levels of iron paired with the inflammation, the doctor ordered more blood tests, urine tests and even stool tests. I remember my mum taking me straight up to the pathology lab. Having just waited for what seemed like forever in the downstairs waiting room, I was really bored when faced with an even more bland room upstairs.

As I'm now recounting the experience in pathology, my memories have started to become a blur, a mix of the dozen times I had tests done there in the months preceding my diagnosis. I now held a card in my hand with a number on the front like I was lining up for the deli section of a supermarket. The card was the only hopeful part of the dull waiting room, my ticket to freedom. As the numbers called started to get close to mine, I could feel the excitement mounting. It is truly something when the most exciting part of your day is waiting to be called up to a pathology appointment.

When my moment to get the blood test taken finally came, I was so relieved. Thankfully, blood tests don't usually take too long. However, I hadn't prepared to give a urine sample because I had quite literally gone to the toilet a half hour prior, which meant that we were delayed another ten minutes whilst I tried to pee. Leaving the doctor's office after being cooped up there for so long was quite relieving. Something about the metal chairs and sitting around hopelessly waiting to be called up just didn't appeal to me. Now, I had many tests that were conducted several times in a few weeks during this part of my diagnosis. However, I have thus far not mentioned what it was like to take a stool test. So what I am going to do in the spirit of transparency is detail the experience in the paragraph below in italics, and anyone who wishes to skip over it may. Everyone else, you can read as much or as little of my experience as you would like.

I had never done one of these tests before, so my mum took it upon herself to reassure me that it was no big deal. If you told me that I was just a month or so away from a cancer diagnosis, I probably would have agreed with her. Despite this, at the time, I was a bit more conflicted. The anticipation of preparing to have to use the bathroom was beginning to worry me. My parents had given me an old ice cream tub to 'submit' the stool into. It was one of those three colour packages with white, brown, and pink stripes for vanilla, chocolate, and strawberry ice cream. Whenever I felt anything around my waist, I wondered whether it was time. The first few were only number ones, although, after a couple of hours the moment came. For some reason, this was even more exciting than my name being called up at the doctor's office, but I guess this was different. After collecting the sample in the ice cream tub, it was my job to open up the medical collection equipment, read the instructions as you would a COVID-19 Rapid Antigen Test (RAT), and carefully transfer the sample from the ice cream container to a plastic container with the equipment provided. I would then bag it and pass it to my parents to rush to pathology. I think it's safe to say my little brother Elijah never ate the chocolate ice cream out of that type of tub again!

Despite my countless and often gruelling tests, what soon became apparent was that we seemed no closer to finding the answer to my itch than when we first started. So I was referred to Dr Murphy, a paediatric specialist familiar with the treatment of allergies. Going to his office was no easy task. First, it was a 35-minute drive from our house, not too far from where my aunty lived, so at least we could occasionally visit her and her family around the appointments if there was time.

Driving towards his office for the first time was not one of those situations with extra time on our hands. Instead, we were cutting it down to the wire and were hoping to find a parking spot outside the front of the office. Furthermore, to make things even more complicated, the office was hidden in and amongst a dozen other buildings that all looked alike and just our luck, there were no easy parking spots. My mum was forced to drop me off near the door with only three minutes to spare before our appointment was scheduled to start. Why am I so panicked about being on time for my appointments if doctors are never on time themselves? It's because there's something about me where I like being early to things or, at the very least, not late, to show punctuality and respect. I began pacing down the sidewalk until I came across the building with the number Mum had texted me. Surprisingly, the bolded signage on the door simply stated the address and didn't make it clear whether I was in the right place, but I had surely made it now.

    The passageway I entered after going through the door had other thoughts. I was immediately confronted by a dozen other offices, and I could turn left, right, continue straight, or go upstairs. I tried matching the room office number I had been sent to those around me, mindful that the clock was against me, and I only had two minutes before my appointment was meant to start. The old staircase to my right was calling me. I chose to race up the stairs, my feet banging against the fragile staircase, dashing up and down the hallway through offices, desperate to see a medical one. However, the office numbers on the doors were not getting any closer to the one I needed. Most of the places were closed, giving this eerie sense that I was off-track. Had I entered through the correct door? I couldn't entertain such thoughts, so back downstairs it was. I probably had about a minute until the appointment when I started to go in the right direction with the numbers getting closer to the one I was searching for. In the back of my mind was the thought my parents had ingrained in me from a young age that one should never be late for a doctor's appointment. I looked down the hall and, in the distance, read a sign saying "Dr Murphy". I had made it, and just in the nick of time.

The ~~Worst~~ Best Year

Dr Murphy would likely be my last hope of discovering the itch's cause. One thing that immediately came to my attention was that my doctor seemed more of a comedian than a medical professional. Now, before I proceed to discuss the odd things about the doctor, I must say that if it wasn't for him, I might never have found out that I had cancer until it was a lot later, maybe too late. In a way, I owe everything I have to this man. It is true that many medical professionals played a part in my diagnosis and treatment, from the GPs to the oncologists. Still, it was this doctor's different thinking that helped to catch my cancer. Maybe he was on the spectrum like me; smart minds think alike.

When I stepped foot in his office for the first time my eyes were instantly pulled to the abstract creatures and pictures of random animals that seemed to come straight from the Shutterstock website. What I found entertaining was how he would constantly use your name when he was speaking. For instance, Dr Murphy would say things such as: "Sebastian, when did your itching first occur, Sebastian?" "Sebastian, how bad would you rate your itch on a scale from 1 to 10?" "Sebastian, have you ever noticed, Sebastian, that certain things make the itch go away, Sebastian?" I guess you could call him personable, but who knew someone could make me bored of my own name?

On one of our subsequent trips to see Dr Murphy we were blessed to not be in such a rush to get there. Having extra time, we chose to pop in at my aunty's house. My little cousin Sarah was only a couple of years old at this point, so joyful and brimming with life. It was always exciting to see her, especially when I was later diagnosed with cancer because it was like her life was an escape from the darkness around me.

Something that stood out about Dr Murphy's waiting room was the liveliness of it. Don't get me wrong, it was still a boring waiting room, but it managed to be a little more interesting. It had splashes of colour brighter than a children's playground around the office space. This was probably to appeal to his younger demographic of patients as opposed to the elderly ones at the local GP. The doctor requested more and more tests, mainly blood tests, but still, nothing turned up. We then tried isolating food groups and nutrients from my diet to determine an allergy. At one point, my mother thought that it would be a good idea to try and isolate gluten from my diet since I worked in a pizza shop and was exposed to lots of gluten. Let me tell you, the week I spent without gluten was one of the hardest weeks I have ever faced. Honestly, I have the utmost respect for people who are intolerant or allergic to gluten because cutting that out of my diet is something that I hope to never have to do again, especially since half of my diet consists of bread.

Despite this and the countless blood tests after blood tests, the doctors still had found nothing. We had performed nearly every test under the sun after our last appointment with Dr Murphy, and we had been able to rule out most bad illnesses that were relevant to my symptoms. I had been using Telfast since the beginning of my itch with great success, but I now also had a range of other medications to use alongside Telfast. Well, at least that was something but although I had completed test after test and ruled one disease out after the other, what remained lacking was the actual cause of this itch. We began to get up to leave the office with a stack of papers even thicker than an iPhone, loaded wallet, and keys stacked on top of each other, showing every test that had recently been performed on me. It was probably as long as this book you're reading now. As my mother and I were getting up and walking out of Dr Murphy's office for what would likely be the last time, he stopped us and said that as we had not done an ultrasound amongst the millions of other things that we had tested, we should get one done. It couldn't hurt, so we agreed and were off on our way but still uncertain. I couldn't wrap my head around what was happening. Was I always going to be like this? Would this itching be transient? Was I overreacting?

On the way home I started pouring through all the tests in the stack of papers. Complete blood counts, vitamin D levels, autoimmune disease tests, pathogen screens, allergen tests, you name it, I had been tested for it. Initially drawn by both my love of statistics and myself, I was fascinated by the detail in the tests. Everything about me, down to a tee, was in these papers. They were a snapshot of myself, the cells inside me, my overall health, and almost everything you could know about me. My mum told me how my diligence in reviewing the papers made her think that *"you'll make a good doctor"*, which, at the time, I shrugged off, thinking it was just my overly proud mother being her usual self. What perplexed me was that all we had was an allergy to dust and that I was blood type O+. My mum was very confused because she thought that since she and my dad were both A+, I had to be A+, and I think she may have questioned whether or not I was her son very briefly. For those of you who are also wondering, the O blood type is a recessive trait. Thus, the allele can be passed on from generation to generation without being the expressed phenotype. In other words, it skips a generation.

The day of the ultrasound was actually kind of fun. I had to fast in the morning, but the appointment was early so it wasn't a big deal. When the sonographer placed the icy cold gel on my stomach, I couldn't help but feel like I was playing the role of a pregnant woman in a movie. The funny thing was that throughout my cancer journey, this feeling would be replicated as the side effects of many of the chemotherapies mimicked that of a pregnant woman. For instance, vomiting, nausea and fluctuating hormone levels. Then there were follow-up ultrasounds, weird stuff happening to your appetite where you sometimes can't stand the sight of food, and other times, you feel like eating for three, weight gain, and much more. Not to say that all these things happened to me. After the ultrasound, I returned to school as if everything was normal. Recess was wrapping up, and I had maths methods next. The class slowly began assembling outside the classroom filling the narrow hallway as neighbouring classes grouped up, waiting for their teachers to open the door. They were let into their classes one at a time as their teachers arrived, and the bell to start the period soon went.

I also loved bells. They marked where one obstacle ended and a new journey began. Our class was the last one to be let into the classroom as the maths teacher had yard duty. Having lost the first few

The ~~Worst~~ Best Year

minutes of class he was eager to begin quickly and make up for lost time. My maths teacher, one of my favourite teachers, often reminded me of my priest in how he looked and spoke, even starting each class, not yelling at the students to be quiet but calmly saying, "Let us begin". Just like a priest, his life was simple but rewarding. Day in and day out he would impart knowledge on the world around him. As the teacher of the enhanced maths class, he shaped the minds of our world's success stories, not concerned by school politics or power but by the love of what he did. Part of me wondered if I should live such a life, but the thought was fleeting. Innately, I knew that I was destined to challenge myself to new heights, which meant going beyond the classroom. Within seconds of the teacher's address, the class' loud energy was silenced as if we were actually in church, and the lesson could begin.

I liked to sit in the front where no one else sat since it allowed me to take up three desks with all my books and equipment while staying comfortable. As I continued through school, I would often rest my right leg up against the chair next to me and use it to swing back and forth throughout the lesson. Later in the class, after we had been sent off to complete some chapter questions in our workbooks, I opened my computer to get the questions up and upon glancing at my emails, I noticed a recent email from Dad. I quickly opened it since he usually only emails time-sensitive things to my school account. It read: "Can you call me as soon as you get this … tell the teacher that you need to leave urgently." Without hesitation, I sprung out of my seat. I shoved the computer with the email opened in my teacher's face, tentatively saying, "Sir, I think I have to go". He told me that it was okay and that I should do what I needed to do.

It turned out that it was for a CT scan, so, as per the notification from my dad, I was picked up at the lunch bell, and then I was back for more tests. The drive over to the screening centre felt a little redundant. I was only there a few hours earlier; it would have been great if we could have done the CT scan then as well. However, I know that would have required them to read my scans on the spot to know I needed the second test, which wasn't very practical. When we arrived at the scanning facility, I was told to drink a litre of a water-like substance in 45 minutes. I might be a fan of water but even that was a lot for my bladder in one sitting. I remember they told me to pace myself over the 45 minutes, which wasn't easy because it meant drinking at a plodding and unnatural pace. Still, sure enough, I tried to maintain a schedule.

It worked out that I needed to drink about one plastic cup per ten minutes. From the outset, I stuck close to my schedule, glancing up at the TV for a scene and then taking a minuscule sip from a tiny plastic cup. I was so bored that I started calculating the amount I would need to sip every 30 seconds to stay on track. It wasn't helpful that the TV was playing mundane daytime shows meant for boring people with no lives and no Netflix subscription. I was far more entertained by the stale-tasting cups of water I was drinking than the tiny TV screen at the end of the waiting room. After a few of these drinking cycles I started to lose my consistency, drinking faster at times and then slower at others until I was finished.

The ~~Worst~~ Best Year

Entering the CT scan room, I had many expectations from the eclectic mix of medical TV shows I had previously seen; to the TV shows' credit, the real deal looked pretty similar. One thing I didn't like was the gown that they made you wear. Don't get me wrong, I understand in surgeries why it's important to have a gown that can easily be taken off, but for a CT scan? If I had a medical emergency, they weren't going to cut me open in the clinic, were they? So why on earth did I need to have the horrid gown on? It wasn't like I was dripping with metal either, or really needed to change! Despite my reservations, I did appreciate the need for consistency and caution, although, to this day, I feel like the gowns could have an updated version for the CT room at least.

The person running the images paced around, casting the impression that they wanted to hurry along the scan and move on with their day, just like me. Having not done a CT scan before, Mum had briefed me on everything to be prepared for. What I found surprising was her thoughts on the side effects of the contrast substance they use. Apparently, it makes you feel as though you have peed yourself even though you actually haven't, which was interesting. She also mentioned that no one told her about this the first time she had the IV contrast, and she had this side effect. Thinking she had peed in her pants, I imagine she may have benefited from all of the deep breathing the machine makes you do during the scan. I also thought it was interesting how the machine talks to you and how some machines use pre-recorded messages instead of someone telling you what to do live. I was definitely grateful for not having the perceived self-urination sensation and I felt pretty good

Sebastian - The Itch

after the scan. It was a quick change in the changing rooms, back into some proper clothes, and I was good to go.

Later that night, I was doing my homework as I usually would when Dad came down the hall and entered my room. "They found something on your scan. It might be cancer. Just like the one Mum had." I could hear the trepidation in his voice and I knew he was trying to keep it together. You could hear a pin drop on the soft carpet in my room. Immediately, I got rid of Dad so I could be alone. I remember when he left, I sat there, his words repeating in my head, unsure of what to think. This soon led to pacing up and down my room trying to make sense of what was happening, and then throwing myself on my bed in frustration. It didn't feel right, so I got back up and looked in the mirror. My reflection was blurry, marred by the dirty handprints on its surface that had accumulated over time. I couldn't see myself clearly, nor the tears gathering in my eyes. Nevertheless, I couldn't let the tears drop; I had to be strong. I had spent my whole life searching for certainty and knowledge, but there was no telling what was next.

Later, post-treatment, I would go on to think about what if I were to have cancer again, and I was upset about the burden I would impose on others around me, the inconvenience of it. However, at the time, having only just been diagnosed with cancer, part of me worried about dying. It was brief, but I thought about what it would be like if the diagnosis was confirmed, and cancer got the best of me. I knew it was unlikely to be the case, but it called a lot into question about me and how I had gone about living. I spent so much of my life thinking about

The ~~Worst~~ Best Year

and preparing for my future, but what if I didn't get a future? What if my life stopped at the young age of 15 and I never reached my full potential? Something within me couldn't shake the thought that I had many more experiences with my loved ones that were owed to me. I was too young to die.

Chapter 5

The Diagnosis

~ *Sebastian*~

I am sure all of you reading this have your own stereotypical idea of what finding out you have cancer is about, and maybe some have experienced what cancer was like for you or a loved one. For me, cancer was a shock but an intriguing one where reassurance triumphed over my nerves. Sure, it was an adjustment for me, and more than a little to take in. Still, I can honestly say that after hearing I had lymphoma, I felt relief above any other emotion since I finally had the answers that I had been so desperately searching for. Any distant thoughts about the danger of treatment not working were mostly subdued. I finally knew why I was itching, meaning I could do something about it which was the important thing.

Despite this, my first appointment at the oncologist's office was a little confronting. The colourful paint on the walls did not match the mood of the emotionless room. Sure, it may have appealed to families that passed through. However, this place was surrounded by people on the verge of death, and the decorated cancer ward was so overfilled with promise. Seeing all those children without any hair and cables coming in and out of their bodies was daunting for someone who, up until a week ago, was living a relatively normal life. I had brought along some schoolwork to complete whilst I was waiting for the doctor. Initially, I was filled with anticipation like I was waiting for an overblown balloon to pop. However, after waiting close to an hour to see the doctor, the air in my balloon soon escaped. I found myself bored out of my mind with nothing else to do but watch as I was surrounded by a half dozen children who were well on their way into chemo and who looked a lot sicker than I did.

My family decided to go downstairs so we didn't spend the whole hour in the waiting room. There was a hospital cafe at the bottom of the elevators straight ahead from where you exited on the way out from the cancer ward. Anything to get away from the cancer ward sounded good to me at the time. The cafe had one of those windows with all the refrigerated foods on offer. A thick piece of caramel slice was beckoning me, so I asked Dad to get one while he bought some coffees. A similar feeling to when my mum was diagnosed permeated my mind that things were about to change. "You know you're not going to end up like those kids in there?" Mum told me. She was eager to keep me calm, and outwardly I was. In some ways that proved to be true, as I maintained a bright and cheerful energy throughout my journey; however, it seemed like the typically bald cancer look was inevitable. I

Sebastian - The Diagnosis

felt an affinity with the bland white walls of the food court because the food court was honest. After all, it was a hospital, a place of dullness. In contrast, the bright decorations of the cancer ward were almost overcompensating, masking the sadness and death that laid within.

When the time finally came for our doctor to see us, I was pleased that I had answers to my itching. The doctor assigned to me seemed friendly and helpful in explaining the situation to my parents and me. At the time, the doctors had yet to make an official diagnosis. They were able to show us the results from the scans that I had already taken, which suggested that I had Hodgkin lymphoma. This would later be confirmed with a PET scan and a core biopsy, where I would learn that I had stage IVA Nodular sclerosis classical Hodgkin lymphoma (NScHL). Long story short, I had cancer which had developed into stage four, meaning that it had spread throughout many parts of the body. This included my spleen, various lymph nodes in my chest and approaching my neck, around the lungs, and bone regions of my lower body. Despite the scary-sounding diagnosis, it was comforting to hear that my condition was still very treatable.

The oncology fellow, Claira, started by asking the usual questions, such as a family history of cancer. We gave them the rundown about my mum, and also a couple of other family members who had suffered from this disease. This may have come as a little bit of a surprise to Claira and the senior oncologist Dr Quinn, since there is minimal evidence suggesting hereditary links to Hodgkin lymphoma. It was one of the not-so-common cancers out there. The doctor now had to feel around to see if she could find any lymph nodes in the armpits, groin, stomach, and more. She was unable to though since the lymph nodes that were inflamed were positioned in the chest where it was more challenging for the doctors to feel for them. Despite having stage IV cancer, from the outside, I was a healthy boy. This was one of the reasons why it was so hard to make the initial diagnosis. Likewise, I felt like a healthy boy, minus the itch, rash and a recent cold. Up until now, I had minimal symptoms indicating my sickness, so coming to terms with just how sick I was, was a challenge. Looking back, I can remember some unexplained temperatures in the lead-up to my diagnosis with a cough that lingered from a respiratory illness I had at the time. On their own, the symptoms didn't seem like much, especially given how vague they were. I was coughing because I had a prolonged sickness two weeks prior. I had a temperature around that time for the same reason, so it was out of my mind. Such a cold probably came at one of the worst times it could have, masking the cause of the temperature for a couple of weeks.

    I felt it strange that we spent so long in the room with the oncologists Dr Claira and Dr Quinn. We were there for what felt like an eternity, and this wasn't the only long session we had with them. The extended visit started to justify why there could often be wait times at the Royal Children's Hospital (RCH) to see doctors, even for scheduled appointments. From my perspective, I don't hold it against the hospital or doctors since they do such a great job at helping as many people as possible in a short time. I do wish there was more support in areas such as oncology across all hospitals, where a few extra doctors could help

Sebastian - The Diagnosis

keep up with increasing demand and streamline the treatment even further for those who cannot afford to be waiting long to see a doctor.

After my family and I arrived home, there was an instant and detectable shift in the attitude and behaviour of everyone around me.

"Do you want a hot chocolate?"

"No, thank you."

"What about a blanket? Are you cold?"

"I'm okay."

"Is there some food I can make you or someplace you want to go?"

The bombardment of support from everyone around me was the opposite of what I was looking for. All I wanted was normality, but the day was as normal as it would get for a 15-year-old boy being diagnosed with cancer. I was still me; I was still the same person, but I felt as though everyone had forgotten that, which made me feel different. Everyone was suddenly extra careful around me. They would pay me extra attention and offer to do things for me that I could very well do myself. Everyone wanted me to know that they were there for me, and the best way they knew how to do that was to offer their help, but in doing this, they made me feel different; they made me feel like I was a new person. I could no longer be Sebastian, the academic genius who everyone loves. I was Sebastian, the kid with cancer, the kid that needed special attention. This was a trend that remained consistent throughout my journey with cancer. Every time I told someone about my cancer, they were initially shocked, as you could imagine, and then they were sympathetic.

The ~~Worst~~ Best Year

I remember when I told one particular friend of mine about my cancer, and they looked at me as if I were a stray, homeless puppy. They gave me that notorious head tilt that people give you when they want you to know they feel sorry for you. No matter what I did or who I told, everyone else saw me as someone who was sick, someone who was impaired. This made the journey through cancer harder since I take great pride in who I am, and for people to see me as nothing more than a sick kid was damaging to that pride. Nevertheless, I held no resentment towards these people since, at the end of the day, their looks of sympathy came from a place of love and compassion. While I found this challenging to deal with, I also felt flattered and loved knowing that everyone else cared for me enough to demonstrate such compassion.

The night after my first appointment at the hospital, I decided to go to work. My environment at the pizza shop was far from the most relaxing. I felt that sometimes my boss was not the most understanding man in the world, but he was still respectable. Although the shop I worked at was owned by a Lebanese family just like my own, the parents of my boss would watch over us like hawks when we worked. This often led to emotions running high in the shop and people getting very upset with one another over pizza orders. Brutal on any random day and dangerous in a fragile emotional state. Because the owners were Lebanese and had a loose connection to my family, I would refer to the parents of my boss as 'Uncle' and 'Aunty' out of respect for them.

On this particular day, my boss' father seemed a little on edge and was telling off many of the workers. For some reason, he kept finding

Sebastian - The Diagnosis

things to tell me off for, and I wasn't too impressed because I was doing my best to help a dozen workers in a tiny, cramped, busy kitchen who all seemed to need my help. I had the pizza makers needing cheese, customers pouring through the front to collect and pay for pizzas, phones ringing non-stop, and customers waiting who needed attention so their orders weren't accidentally forgotten about. All of this whilst I was dodging and weaving through a tiny kitchen with way too many people in it and trying to help everyone simultaneously meant that some things took time. Unfortunately, my boss' father wasn't too happy with this, but all I could say was, "Sorry, Uncle", and move on. Throughout this busy part of the night, he grew increasingly upset with me, which made me equally, if not more upset with him. Eventually, as I went to the freezer to get cheese for the pizza makers, he got angry with me for not staying at the front more to take care of the million other things simultaneously and leaving it to my other co-workers.

Throughout the shift, this began to eat away at me and I took a moment to just let out what I was feeling. This was my first chance to let out a tear and let others know about what was happening, while thinking about the journey ahead. I was in a state of confusion, unsure of whether I should be scared, excited, or calm. All I knew was that I needed a moment to work things out for myself. Just my luck, one of my coworkers was coming out of the back office and she saw me. Visibly surprised by my emotion, she tried to comfort me, but it was no use. "Are you alright?" I didn't know what to say, so I just said: "It looks like I have cancer." She offered her affection and hugs, but my emotions were too intense to care. I liked knowing that no matter what happened, I would be supported, which instilled within me all the confidence I needed. One of my mum's cousins happened to work with me at the pizza shop, and he was next to find out. As he was walking out towards the back of the shop, he noticed my emotional state and asked what happened.

"The doctors reckon I have Hodgkin lymphoma."

"What's that?"

"Cancer. They're going to do some more tests to confirm, but it looks like I have cancer."

It had been a while since the C-word struck our family, but it had come and wasn't going away soon. Within a minute or so, I had half of the shop drop what they were doing to come and check in on me. Ironic given this thing started when my boss' father tried to keep everyone working, and now, the whole shop's productivity was dropping. It felt nice being supported by the others working at the shop, knowing they had my back.

It was getting towards the back end of my shift, so given the circumstances, my boss let me go home early. I walked out the front of the shop with everyone on my side, ready to give me anything I needed. My boss' sister came out to check on me while I was waiting for my dad to pick me up. He was at my Aunty Monique's house as my family was visiting them while I was at work. My boss' sister was the most understanding and sympathetic of the owners' family. If something was wrong, she would know, and you could feel reassured, leaving it to her

Sebastian - The Diagnosis

to fix things. While she couldn't cure my cancer, she did what she could to support me, and that was all I could ask for from her. My boss' sister seemed interested in what would happen to me and would frequently check in over the course of my treatment, even after I stopped working at the pizza shop; for that, I am nothing but grateful.

The boss' father must have been saddened about how we left things and offered me a free pizza. I chose to get the lot. I didn't usually, although I did like to mix things up with my choices. A short while back, the workers would be given a free pizza at the end of each shift, and I made it my mission to try every pizza on our menu. I guess it helped me to handle customers who asked what the nicest pizzas were and what kind of pizza I thought they might like based on their tastes. Plus, it was fun to try different things and set myself goals. Unfortunately, the workers were not allowed to do this anymore as free pizzas for everyone was not sustainable, however, that night was my lucky exception.

My pizza came out in only a few minutes, and not long after, my dad was pulling up to the shop, so I was off. "Mum and your brothers are visiting Aunty Monique's family if you want to join, or you could go home and rest." My parents were eager to make sure that I wasn't tiring myself out and that I was feeling okay, so I often told them I was good. This way, they were happy and I didn't have to hear them panicking. If something was really wrong, I would tell them when I needed to, but telling my parents anything else felt like I was taking unnecessary attention and spreading excess fear. That night, I figured I could use the distraction, so I told Dad to take me to see them. The drive over was pretty silent. I filled the silence digging into the pizza in my hands.

Their house was only a couple of minutes from the pizza shop, so the drive of silence didn't last long. Walking in, I knew the attention was going to be on me. I was now fundamentally different in the eyes of everyone around me, and I was going to be seen as the special kid with cancer for the next six months, so I thought I'd better start getting used to it. This specialness, I didn't mind. I liked to feel special so long as I was still treated like a healthy person where practical.

Everyone seemed excited to see me. I also now had the chance to properly dig into the pizza. "What's that?" Mum asked. She knew workers were not allowed free pizzas anymore. Having just told my dad they gave me the pizza for free, he told her, "The boss' old man gave it to him". His surprised tone fit perfectly since the boss' dad was known to spend his cash wisely, and it meant even more that he had given me the pizza because of it. Back when I got a free pizza at the end of each shift it didn't mean as much, but now, I savoured the pizza and it felt more special. After eating, I went upstairs to make a call. I had just told my entire workplace about my diagnosis, and it was time to tell my closest friends, Zac and Connor.

"Connor, I have something to tell you."

"Yeah."

"It looks like I have Hodgkin lymphoma."

"That's cancer, isn't it?"

"Yeah."

"Is this a joke?"

Sebastian - The Diagnosis

"No, why?"

What I didn't realise was that when I called him, it was April 1st, and so understandably, he thought I was playing some elaborate April Fools' Day joke on him. When I confirmed that I was serious, his mood suddenly plummeted. "Are you okay? If you need anything, I'm here." We continued like this for a little while, and then I rang Zac. By the "Oh shit" Zac gave me, he was no less surprised. It made sense to ask them to keep things under wraps for the moment whilst I was waiting for the confirmation of diagnosis, and then getting around to telling anyone else I wanted to personally.

I started to imagine what it would be like with the roles reversed, if I was the one having a close friend call out of the blue and tell me they have cancer. When you're in survival mode, you often are immune to the magnitude of what you are dealing with. It's only on rare occasions that you say to yourself, "Oh shit, I have cancer!" You realise how much you have changed. It was weird for me to think about what it would be like if a 15-year-old mate of mine made that call to me, and I couldn't help but sympathise with my friends, which might sound crazy, but I hope it can make sense to even a few of you. In the coming days, when my diagnosis was confirmed, the wider community became aware of my situation, and I was being supported by anyone and everyone who had even heard the name Sebastian Khoury.

It wasn't long before I received a Positron Emission Tomography (PET) scan and Magnetic Resonance Imaging (MRI) to confirm the staging of my cancer. On the day of my joint PET-MRI scans, I remember entering the hospital without having fully comprehended what was happening to me. In the limited time since my initial ultrasound, I had switched to survival mode. I had blocked out the worries of cancer and was only focused on my recovery.

Before we could reach the imaging department, Mum and I faced some hurdles. The primary one was limited parking. This meant that unless you had an early appointment, you were unlikely to find a spot easily. Luckily, our appointment was outside peak hours, although we weren't always so fortunate. With one hurdle cleared, it was on to the COVID-19 check-in. It was 2022, but the world of the RCH had yet to forget the pandemic. When entering the ground floor from the elevator, you were greeted by four queues to enter your details and receive an identification sticker from the front desk. Making dozens of people stand in multi-rowed lines together for ten minutes indoors was probably not the most effective way to stop COVID spreading, but that didn't stop the hospital. I guess it gave people a sense of security and safety from illness. When you're visiting loved ones who are sick in the hospital, a bit of reassurance isn't too bad.

Often, my mum would spend a lot of time analysing which line had the most momentum, which might have saved us some time. Sometimes, if the lines were long and we were looking to get out of the lines quickly, we would end up in two different queues and then move together into the same line once it was clear who had the better one. On occasion, if our line wasn't cutting it, we would go under the belt dividing the lines so that we could get checked in and to our appointment faster.

Sebastian - The Diagnosis

However, today was a clear run. A mere two people stood in front of us in the queue, and we were checked in within no time.

The lower ground floor of the RCH was the home of medical imaging. This is where you would receive a PET, MRI, Computed Tomography (CT) scan and much more. People of all shapes and sizes, from infancy to late teens, would end up in this place for a myriad of potential causes, such as a broken arm or, in some cases akin to mine, cancer. After a short while of boredom, Mum and I were called into the room to prepare for the PET-MRI scan. One of the medical staff looking after me was Montanna. She explained what the scans would entail and the reasons for them. As one might expect, I was asked about metal implants and jewellery that I had on me.

For the PET scan to be effective, it needed to determine which parts of my body were metabolically active. This would allow radiologists and oncologists to determine what parts of my body the cancerous cells had spread to, as these cells would be metabolically active. To assist with the clarity of the scan, a cannula was inserted in my right arm that would allow the medical staff to efficiently and safely inject contrast intravenously. Moreover, I was given medication to make me tired so as to make the experience more comfortable. I then spent the next 30-45 minutes watching *The Italian Job* while I waited for the contrast to spread throughout my body. During this time, I once again didn't fully appreciate the magnitude of what I was going through. Despite grappling with a life-threatening illness, my body had prioritised surviving, so much so that cancer and the risks of its progression were some of the last things

The ~~Worst~~ Best Year

on my mind. Instead, I focused on scans and treatment.

Inside the room where the scan was conducted, I was instructed to remove my mask and lie down on a flat, cushioned table. Within no time, I was being strapped into the machine decked out with belts, buckles and straps akin to a prototype of a superhero outfit. Inside the machine, I had the luxury of watching the same movie from earlier. However, this time it was hardly the Gold Class cinema experience over the thumping loud bangs and doof-doofs of the scanning machinery. It was like police sirens were constantly going off in my head. I would surely get some hearing loss from such deafening thumps if I did enough of these.

My mother, hesitant to leave her 15-year-old son in the room alone, decided to stick around as much as she could. I am not sure whether she thought she was doing it to calm me or herself, but it didn't hurt anyone having her there since I didn't see her anyway. I was to look straight up in the rectangular mirror above my head, which was angled to capture the reflection of a TV in the opposite direction, with sound being pumped through the headphones on my ears. In between thumps, I could hear the background music of the movie and short dialogue, interrupted by bangs louder than the drums of a Lebanese wedding. It was enough to get the jist of what was happening and distract my mind. After a near two hours of the machine's pounding, the tests were finally over. I was allowed to go down to the food court for lunch and enjoy the rest of my day.

The lunch area may have been small, but it had enough. There were your basics: McDonald's, cafes and a mix of East Asian cuisine.

Sebastian - The Diagnosis

The trinity of food court essentials. After all, could it really be a food court if the kids couldn't get McDonald's, or the parents couldn't get their caffeine fix? It also wouldn't be an Australian food court without a multicultural influence, hence the fried rice and chicken in the food warmers. On this particular day, I had McDonald's on my radar, and I was keen to eat following the previous two hours of loud and unpleasant bangs. Montanna told me that in her nine months working at the hospital, she had only managed to go to Maccas once. Still, I felt as though I had earned the right to eat some fries after my pain, and thus, I scored a guilt-free lunch at McDonald's. After getting my food, my nose was filled with the scent of freshly cooked fries, and my stomach was calmed by the meal that it had been waiting for all morning. But my euphoria was short-lived. Mum soon received news that one of the scans was not of adequate clarity and parts needed to be repeated, so my lunch would have to wait a while longer. Following another half-hour delay, I was finally free to dig into my lunch, and I could be rewarded for my long day of hunger.

The next appointment with Quinn and Claira was the chance to discuss the contents of the scans. My parents and I were formally told about what regions in my body were impacted by cancer and discussions were had about how the diagnosis would be confirmed with a core biopsy of the chest lymph nodes. They told us what treatment for Hodgkin's would look like, giving us pamphlets about doxorubicin, etoposide, vincristine, and prednisolone. Collectively, these would form part of an 'OEPA' treatment against Hodgkin lymphoma. One thing that stuck out was that Claira mentioned etoposide could predispose me to leukaemia in the future. My mum jumped on this with concern, but Claira explained to her that "our job is to focus on the cancer that we are currently faced with and deal with the rest if it comes to that".

Again, sitting through a one-hour session with the doctor may have seemed excessive, but I found it enjoyable. As much as it was hard to see my journey through cancer from a doctor's perspective, it is pretty interesting to consider what it would be like in Quinn's and Claira's shoes, looking at a 15-year-old whose life was just turned upside down and making decisions to get him through his troubles so he could survive cancer. Since having been the beneficiary of their help, I have felt an even closer interest in medicine than before diagnosis and I am truly motivated to do for others what my oncologists could do for me.

Chapter 6

This Can't Be Happening Again

~ Natalie ~

You don't know that you have lived your worst day until you do. There have been times in my life when I thought I had experienced my worst day. We have all been there at some point or another. How many times have you said: "This was the worst day of my life!" You may believe you have lived your worst day at a particular time, but there can always be an even worse day. I never thought this was possible after my cancer diagnosis in 2013, but for me, this day occurred on Thursday, 31st March 2022.

It started months before when my middle child, Sebastian, developed an itch. It was not severe initially, but it became more intense over time. After Sebastian had received his COVID vaccine, he developed chest pains and so began the process of elimination through a series of tests. You may be thinking *he had an itch just like her, so they should have known*. Back in 2013, 'itchiness' was one of my symptoms. However, eight years on, cancer didn't even cross our minds! For Sebastian, the itch was all over his body. We were going through a pandemic, and a new vaccine was being administered, a vaccine that we were still learning about its side effects. A few days after his first vaccination for COVID-19, Sebastian woke up with chest pains. We found ourselves back at the same clinic where I was diagnosed eight years earlier, seeing a doctor we had never seen before. Dr Brenda had left many years prior and over the years, we had been seeing random doctors at this clinic. The young doctor we had an appointment with ran some tests that showed some elevated inflammation markers, and he was not too concerned with the chest pain as the tests that were conducted all came back clear. So we left it at that. Luckily, a knock on Sebastian's head a couple of months later brought us back to the clinic to see Dr Lillian. I mentioned to her that his previous blood tests had elevated inflammation markers, and she said she would like to investigate that further. Sebastian would tell you that Dr Murphy saved his life when he discovered his cancer. I agree with that, but if it weren't for Dr Lillian, the process of eliminating why he had an itch would not have started.

Dr Lillian wanted to know why his inflammation markers were still elevated. She did not ignore the symptoms! I believe it was a great medical team that found this cancer. Dr Lillian checked for everything, including Crohn's disease, liver function, kidney function, thyroid, and coeliac just to name a few, and they all came back clear. She even checked different cancer markers and was pleased that the results came back clear. Nothing could explain the inflammation and the itching

Natalie - This Can't Be Happening Again

that Sebastian was experiencing, so she recommended that we see a paediatrician. It was never a simple process. She wrote a referral to the paediatrician my boys used to see when they were babies. When I rang to book an appointment, I was told he had retired. We were out to dinner with a friend who recommended a doctor on his side of town who specialises in allergies. When I arranged the new referral to see this doctor, it was almost Christmas, and all the clinics were closed for the holidays. We did not get in with Dr Murphy until January. Elijah tested positive for COVID on the day of the appointment. Back then, if one family member tested positive for COVID, the whole household had to be isolated for a week, meaning our appointment was pushed out to mid-February.

When we walked in, Dr Murphy commented on Dr Lillian's expertise, as she had not left much for him to test for. He requested more blood tests to see if anything showed up. During the last visit, Dr Murphy informed us that there was nothing more he could test for. He wanted us to keep an allergy diary to see what Sebastian ate whenever this itch occurred. We were literally walking out the door, but my gut was telling me something was wrong. Earlier that week, I found Sebastian napping in the afternoon, which he had never done. We were almost out the door when Dr Murphy asked us to come back into his office as there was one more test he wanted us to do. We were literally walking out! This could have easily continued for another couple of months back and forth, tracking Sebastian's diet, but someone up in Heaven was watching over us. Dr Murphy requested an ultrasound of the abdomen.

The ~~Worst~~ Best Year

I asked him what he was looking for, and he informed us that kidney and liver function could show different things in an ultrasound than a simple blood test.

When we entered the clinic for the ultrasound, the sonographer enquired why we were having this ultrasound done. I explained to her that Sebastian had an intense itch that would not ease. She said a "great medical team" would be doing this ultrasound based on the symptoms I had explained. This ultrasound was the final examination that ultimately found the cancer located in his spleen. We completed the test the morning of March 31st. I knew by the look on the sonographer's face that she had found the cause of his symptoms. Although she couldn't disclose what she had found, she advised us that we would get an answer before the end of that day. I tried to remain positive and assured Sebastian that we would soon find out what was causing the itching. Inside, I felt anxious and nervous. Deep down my intuition knew that the news would be bleak.

Within an hour, I received a phone call from the receptionist at the doctor's office informing us that we would need to take Sebastian back to get an urgent CT scan that same day. He was not to eat anything, and the radiography place would call us soon. They rang me immediately and said to bring him down at 1.00 pm for the CT scan. I picked him up from school and remained calm for him, but I felt like I was about to fall apart. We did not arrive home from the scan until 3.00 pm. I called the receptionist at Dr Murphy's office as soon as we were done to see how long it would take to receive the results. He was out of the office, but she would call him on his mobile as soon as the results were in. I received that call from Dr Murphy an hour and a half later. He enquired after George to ensure that he was with me. My stomach sank. George and I went into the study to take the call, and I put the phone on speaker.

Dr Murphy was compassionate and kind. He spoke slowly and explained that he suspected Sebastian had Hodgkin lymphoma. He informed us that it was quite advanced as it had spread to multiple areas in his body. He had spoken to the Children's Hospital, and a fellow (a trainee specialist) from the hospital would be calling us soon, as we may have to visit the hospital that night or the following morning. In that moment I experienced that out-of-body experience I spoke about earlier. As George spoke with the doctor, I no longer heard the words spoken, and I can recall punching my fist into the couch countless times as we sat in the study and repeating the word "NO" over and over.

How can this be happening to us yet again? We had already experienced our turn of bad luck. This boy was planning to top his grades to achieve an ATAR (Australian Tertiary Admissions Rank) to be able to study dentistry and was looking for work experience to support his goal. He loved his part-time job at the pizza shop and enjoyed playing tennis. Having cancer was not in his plan. This was not going to be his year, and it did not matter how much I wished it not to be true; the reality was that it was true. This was every parent's nightmare. My child had cancer, and all the power I had as a parent was gone. I could no longer control anything that was going to happen.

Thank God for George at that moment. We knew we had to tell

The ~~Worst~~ Best Year

Sebastian immediately, but we needed to get our emotions under control. I felt like someone had their hands around my throat, and I could not breathe; I wanted to be sick. George sat with me until I stopped hyperventilating, and then what started flowing were just pure, raw tears that did not dissipate. George said he would speak to Sebastian as I would most likely scare him if he saw me in that state. I do not know what he said to Sebastian or how he even could explain these words to our son, but he did. George is the strongest person I know. I cannot even begin to fathom the difficulty of looking into your child's eyes and saying those words.

While George was in Sebastian's room, I went into Jerome's room and told him. I had no idea how to tell Jerome that his brother had cancer. I informed him that we had just spoken to Dr Murphy. Jerome knew by the look on my face, and in between my tears, I shared with him that his brother Sebastian had what I once had. I just could not say the words that Sebastian had cancer. I saw Jerome's heartbreak. He was getting ready to go to work. I should have waited until he had finished work to tell him. I didn't even think about it, but I knew I couldn't drive him to work at that point. I asked him to call in sick as I could not drive him in, but he insisted he didn't want to miss his shift. He needed to be out of the house. My beautiful friend Angela had been calling me all day to get updates, so I rang her and asked if she could take Jerome to work for me. This lady is a saint. You know that friend you can always rely on; they just know what you need. Angela is a pure angel and the perfect example of an amazing friend.

Natalie - This Can't Be Happening Again

The next phone call I had to make was going to be just as heartbreaking. I called my mother. I spoke sternly and told her I needed her to be my mother, to remain strong despite what I was about to disclose to her, and not to fall apart. She began to panic and asked, "Natalie, you are scaring me. What is wrong?" My mother panicked at the best of times. I shared the devastating news with her and asked her to remain strong. Then the shared tears flowed between the two of us. She kept repeating, "Not Sebastian, not Habibi (my darling) Sebastian". She told me she was coming over. I told her she needed to calm down first. I wanted to make sure she was calm before she drove the car. She reassured me she would be okay with driving.

I walked into Sebastian's room to check in on him once I had gained control of my tears. He was sitting quietly at his desk completing schoolwork. My immediate thoughts were how was he functioning after the news he had just received to be doing schoolwork. Later on I would discover that it was in fact the schoolwork that kept him grounded and helped him remain focussed throughout his ordeal. He looked calm, which unsettled me. He was not easy to read at the best of times. I needed to know that he was okay. He assured me that he was fine. I told him that if he had any questions I was there to answer them, reminding him that I had been through a similar experience. He was short with me and replied, "Mum, I said I am fine". So I left the room.

From there, I found refuge in my front garden, where I sat on the cold concrete step and cried my heart out. At that moment, I just wanted to hold him and tell him it would be okay. The hard truth is that nobody really knew the outcome except God. I wanted to take the cancer out of his body and put it back into mine.

Angela came to pick up Jerome for work, but George had already driven him by this time, so she sat with me and held me while I cried. Then my mother arrived. I could not look at her. I knew how much she loved Sebastian. She always said she didn't have favourites when it came to her grandchildren, but she had a soft spot for him. Angela went and hugged my mother while she cried. I could not hug my mother because I knew that if I did, I would feel all her pain too. I was not coping with my pain as it was and couldn't take her pain as well.

Angela and I worked together and were meant to work together that evening. She has been a part of our family for many years, but she put her grief aside to support me. Angela organised to have all of my work shifts cancelled indefinitely so I could concentrate solely on the steps needed to be taken for my son to be healthy once more. My mother went inside to see Sebastian, holding it together for him. I knew it was killing her to speak to him without crying but she did. I had warned her before we went in not to cry as I didn't want to scare him. She stayed for a bit then went home. Her support was what I needed.

Lanelle and Monique, my two closest friends, were waiting to hear the outcome of the scans. I do not have sisters, but these two women have been a part of my life since I was a baby; they are my sisters. I could not answer their calls as I couldn't speak. Their concerns were evident with their incessant ringing, so I sent them a text explaining that I couldn't talk. They knew this meant we had received the results. Lanelle

Natalie - This Can't Be Happening Again

sent a message "I'm coming over". I rang her, and in between my tears, I told her not to come as I did not want Sebastian to feel overwhelmed. She suggested that we go over to her house so Sebastian could hang out with her children and George and I could have a moment to come to terms with it all. I can't recall if I shared the news with her, but she knew it wasn't favourable. We went over to Lanelle and her husband Joseph's home. Monique, her husband Joe and her family met us there. It was just what we needed because Sebastian and Elijah were outside playing with the children, and George and I were able to let out our grief with our closest friends. Sebastian was the only child amongst them who knew the heartbreaking news, so it was a welcomed distraction.

At 7.00 pm, before we had left for Lanelle and Joseph's house, I had received a call from the Royal Children's Hospital (RCH). It was the fellow that would be looking after Sebastian. Her name was Claira, and she sounded so compassionate. She answered the list of questions that I had already put together. Dr Claira said Sebastian would need to present to the oncology ward at the RCH in the morning. I could not believe we were having this discussion. It was a Thursday night, and at 8:30 am in the morning we had been doing a routine ultrasound. Now, we were in the process of booking oncology appointments. What was going on? I felt like it was a nightmare. Seriously, think about it: you wake up to take your child to a routine ultrasound, and then that same day, you go to bed crying your heart out because your child has cancer. That night, I went into the shower so I could cry without anyone hearing me. It was a long shower, and I cried until I could no longer stand. I then sat on the floor of the shower in despair. I did not come out until George came and took me out. I have no idea how long I was in there, but I just remember the water being turned off and George putting a towel around me. It was such a blur.

The next morning George and I took Sebastian to the RCH. With the COVID-19 rules in place at the time, only one parent was allowed in with the child, but Dr Claira, the fellow, received approval for George to come along. Imagine doing this on your own! Thank God she was able to. Walking through those Day Oncology doors was so confronting—not just for us but also for Sebastian. The children in the waiting room looked so sick. I could see the fear in Sebastian's eyes. The receptionist said Claira was stuck in a meeting and suggested we grab a coffee so we went downstairs to the cafeteria. We were there for a while and then I asked Sebastian, "Do you want to go back up?" "Not yet," he replied. He made a comment about being depressed by the sight of all the sick children in the oncology ward. I can't remember his exact words. I told him not to compare himself to the other children. We had no idea what we were facing yet. "Let's wait and see what the doctors tell us." It was difficult, but I tried to remain positive for him.

We headed back to Day Oncology and waited for a while longer. Time passed us by. I approached the receptionist and asked if Dr Claira would be much longer. She said she was not sure. Then I got frustrated. I said, "Do you understand that our anxiety levels are increasing by the minute and a time frame would be nice?" I know it was not her fault but I was really struggling. I thought that going in and seeing the doctor would give me all the answers. Little did I know that was not going to be the case. Five minutes after my outburst, Claira called us in.

She was just as amazing as I had imagined her to be, a young doctor who coincidentally was from our side of town. She started to build a lovely rapport with Sebastian. When I pulled out my pink diary with my long list of questions, she answered them as best she could. She called in Dr Quinn, the specialist in charge of Sebastian's case. We told Dr Quinn we did not want a different doctor for every visit, or we would choose private treatment for Sebastian. I am so glad we didn't. It is well known that the RCH is one of the best hospitals in the world, and honestly, I can see why. Dr Quinn reassured us that he would be the primary doctor in charge. He told us we would meet with the fellow between appointments, and see him for all the main appointments unless he was unavailable. The way it worked was Dr Quinn and Dr Claira were our doctors, and they were part of a team of seven doctors. They would meet once a week to discuss their cases. If the patient's case was complicated, other doctors would be involved with the care to share ideas on the best course of treatment. Sebastian's case became quite complicated 15 days in. So, I am glad that we decided to stick with this team.

I wished we had walked out of that appointment knowing more, but we had to wait until we did the PET scan and core biopsy. At this point, they suspected it was Hodgkin lymphoma. They thought it was advanced to stage 3, maybe even stage 4. The following Tuesday was the PET scan, and we were hoping that the surgery for a core biopsy could happen the day after that. A core biopsy is when they take a chunk of the cancerous cell out. The ideal outcome would be taking out the whole lymph node. We left the appointment feeling very overwhelmed, with even more questions than answers.

We had not told many people as we were waiting for an official diagnosis, but when we left the hospital, my phone was flooded with missed calls and text messages. Our very close family had heard the news, and so many people who cared about us rang. However, at this point I was feeling like I was drowning. I returned a couple of calls, but it was all too much. I had no answers! People would call me crying, which just triggered my crying. My heart felt like it was going to explode. Friends and family meant well, but their questions at this time didn't help alleviate my anxiety. Our loved ones were concerned but the constant messages and queries about Sebastian's condition were exhausting. I was still processing it all and did not want to accept what was occurring. I was emotionally exhausted. I received messages of support that said, "We are praying for you," or "We are here for you," and such messages provided me with immense comfort. I knew I had countless people who loved us and wanted to be there for us, yet I felt the loneliest I had ever felt. It is the hardest feeling to describe. You are surrounded by so much love, yet you feel so alone.

I kept looking at Sebastian, seeing the confusion in his eyes. We left the hospital late that day, and he told us he wanted to return to work. I wanted his life to stay as normal as possible, so I agreed despite my better judgement. When I dropped him off at work, I spoke to his

Natalie - This Can't Be Happening Again

boss about what was happening and explained that he was not ready to tell anyone. His boss was devastated by the news. He said Sebastian could work when he wanted for however long he wanted. Monique had Elijah at her house after school. Elijah loved hanging out with Monique's children. He called them his cousins, and it was such a blessing to have their support to distract Elijah at this time, as he still did not know what was happening. Monique invited us to wait for Sebastian to finish work at her house. A couple of hours into Sebastian's work shift, he rang us to pick him up. I knew something was wrong. I stayed at Monique's house, and George went to get him. He had become overwhelmed at work and needed to leave. This poor boy was trying to do it all and hold it together. He was doing a fantastic job - even better than we were. It was so heartbreaking. He walked into Monique's house, and I said, "Let's go home." "No, let's stay," he replied, "but I need you to call Aiden (his psychologist) now and make an appointment." I immediately sent an email to Aiden explaining why we needed to see him urgently.

Sebastian had been seeing Aiden for many years for his Autism, and I think this was what gave him the tools to be able to cope the way he did. Sebastian was diagnosed with Autism when he was in Prep. There are so many different levels of Autism. Unfortunately, it is not straightforward for many children going through a diagnosis like Autism, but each child is unique, and every treatment plan is specific to that child. We had put everything we had into any type of therapy to help Sebastian grow and develop. I believe this gave him the strength to deal with what he had to go through. When I was first told Sebastian had

The ~~Worst~~ Best Year

Autism, I thought it was going to stop him from being able to do things in life. I quickly learned that this was a strength and not a weakness. Once I understood how his mind worked, I started to see that he just thought differently from others, which was not a negative thing at all. Knowing he had this allowed us to get him the help to deal with whatever would hold him back. Learning to deal with what was holding him back was what gave him the strength to move forward in life. Although there are different scales of Autism, Sebastian has been able to achieve all his great accolades because of his Autism. Do not get me wrong, it was not smooth sailing. Many obstacles had to be overcome throughout the years. He had to work very hard to overcome so many social barriers growing up. We had to work very hard to overcome our expectations of life being perfect for him to get to where we are today.

  That night at Monique's home, as we sat around her dining table, Sebastian told me it was time to tell his little brother Elijah about his diagnosis. I wanted to wait until we returned home, but Sebastian was adamant that he would be told immediately. Elijah was playing with Monique's son. Sebastian called Elijah over. With Monique sitting at the table beside me, I said, "Elijah, remember when you were a baby and Mum was sick?" With his nod of approval, I went on to explain, "All these tests Sebastian has been undertaking have shown that he has the same disease I had, but he is going to be okay." I continued to tell him that Sebastian had many hospital visits coming up. Elijah instantly replied, "I knew something was going on," and then returned to play. I was relieved by his reaction. I was unsure as to how much he processed. Later that year, I read a piece he wrote at school which gave me an insight into what he was feeling. He actually processed it all but didn't want to show me that emotion.

The next day, Lanelle invited us over for dinner as she had her cousin, an oncologist from Adelaide, visiting. She said it may help to sit and chat with her. It was a privilege to do exactly that with Gabby. I did not know Gabby prior to that evening, but after the dinner I felt like she was one of my good friends. She held my hand and answered my questions. She was careful not to promise anything, but I felt reassured that we had a good chance of fighting this awful disease head-on. My biggest concern was that Sebastian's treatment plan would be very different to my own. After speaking with Gabby, I felt reassured that the doctors were taking us down the right path.

When I returned home that night, I felt like I could breathe a little. The next day, I felt a little stronger and could return some phone calls. I only called back a couple of people at a time though because their crying would trigger my own. I truly felt everyone's love, but I was physically and emotionally drained, and it was only day three.

Chapter 7

Life Goes On, But The Tests Do Not Stop

~ Natalie ~

On Monday, April 4th, four days after finding out the worst news of my life, I woke up in the morning and decided to make a trip to the church so that I could talk with God. I had been so angry all week and questioned my faith after Sebastian's diagnosis. The feeling was so profound that I believed I would never enter a church again. Our family have always been strong practising Catholics. My faith was what helped me through my diagnosis. It helped me through the grief of losing my father, and it strengthened me through other challenging times. This time, I felt that having faith was a waste of time because I was a good person, and my son was an angel. Every time I was faced with an obstacle in life, it usually only made my faith stronger.

This time, I felt that this was the biggest punishment God could have placed upon me. I would yell at God, "Why? Why Sebastian? Why our family?" I would become extremely annoyed when people would say

Natalie - Life Goes On, But The Tests Do Not Stop

God will not give you anything you cannot handle. I thought to myself, *What bullshit, how am I meant to handle this?* I was barely keeping my head above water. I knew the road ahead was going to be gruelling. I honestly didn't know how to get through the next day, let alone the next few months. But when I had time to process it all, I decided to pray and release my anger. My faith was stronger than I realised. I arrived at the church and the doors were closed. There was no Mass on that day so I returned home and said to George, "God must be angry with me after all the things I have been saying... he did not open the doors for me this morning". I never knew that the church closed on Mondays. I thought the church always remained open.

On April 5th, we were scheduled to get the PET scan done. I had time in the morning before the appointment, so I thought I would try my luck and see if God would open his church door for me this time. I really felt the need to go to church and have a chat with God. Like I said earlier, I had been very upset with God up until this point, but I felt a strong urge to go and pray with all my heart. The doors were open, and that was exactly what I did. If you have ever prayed with all your heart, you will know what I mean by that. I felt a sense of calm after my hour of prayer. With my arms open, I prayed the Our Father prayer and felt a warmth come into my heart. At the end of the Mass, I knelt and prayed, speaking with my dad in Heaven and I felt his presence beside me. I honestly felt like he was standing beside me. I felt calm and at peace. After Mass, we made our way to the RCH for Sebastian to have a PET scan.

The ~~Worst~~ Best Year

The PET scan is different to the CT scan. Nothing hides in a PET scan. You are injected with a radioactive dye and must wait an hour in a low-light room for it to take effect. After you do a PET scan, it is recommended that you stay away from young children and pregnant women for six hours. The procedure involves lying down on a bed that then enters into a very loud 'tunnel machine' while images are taken. The sound the machine makes resembles a big thumping drum noise. We were told after the PET scan we would have to do an echocardiogram. This test takes a mapping of the heart, so it would be another long day.

Sebastian did not complain about any of the procedures they asked him to undergo. Fasting was involved, and he just did it. They injected him with the radioactive dye, and we waited in the quiet room watching the movie. He chose to watch *The Italian Job*. When the prescribed amount of time had passed, they took him in for the scan. I remember how loud that machine was when I had mine done, and I remember the emotions I was feeling at the time, so I did not want to leave him alone. I told the nurse I would sit at the back of the machine and go in with him. I could not tell if he could see me, but I needed to be there for him. They told us it would take an hour, but it took closer to two. This made me nervous.

It was 2:20 pm, and Sebastian was very hungry, and groggy as they had given him medication to make him relax before he went in for the scan. We had 40 minutes to grab something to eat before the echocardiogram test on his heart. We went downstairs to McDonalds. I was grabbing a coffee when I bumped into Sebastian's friend and

Natalie - Life Goes On, But The Tests Do Not Stop

his mum. The minute that she enquired about our presence at the hospital, I broke down and started to cry. Again, I collected myself so that Sebastian wouldn't see me in my emotional state. Before we could even begin to enjoy our food, I received a call from the radiology department asking us to return as they needed to take another scan from a different angle. The poor child just wanted to dig into his lunch but had to go back up. As much as I felt bad that he could not have a break, I needed to find out exactly what this beast was, so we did what we needed to do. Sebastian did not complain either. It only took 15 minutes or so, and then he was able to get back to his lunch and then have a heart scan.

When we arrived home that night, you could feel that it was all starting to take a toll on Sebastian's mental state. He was very snappy and frustrated, but who could blame him? He must have been holding in so many emotions. Everything I did seemed to annoy him, and I was trying hard to keep my emotions under wraps. It was not easy. I used to hate when people fussed over me when I had cancer, but he was my child; I just did not know how to give him the space that he needed.

At 6:30 pm, we received a call from Dr Claira, the fellow oncologist, informing us that Sebastian would be on the emergency operations list the following afternoon. She said there was no guarantee it would happen, but he needed to fast, and come in. My anxiety was through the roof, as the past couple of nights Sebastian had been having night sweats, and this was a sign of cancer that was very advanced. Every afternoon, he was taking naps which was understandable given the type of days we were having, and I am sure he was not sleeping that well at night. I just needed to know what we were dealing with.

The following day before we went to surgery, we went to see Dr Claira who informed us that the lumps were too deep. They were hoping to take one out of his neck, but they could not physically feel it. So they decided that they would biopsy the one in his chest. This was more invasive, and it meant we would have to stay overnight to monitor his heart after surgery. If we did the surgery that day, we would have all the results on staging by the following Monday. At 1:00 pm they did a COVID test before surgery and put us in a private room while waiting for the COVID PCR results to come back. At 3:00 pm we were still waiting in the room. It felt like they had forgotten us there. I was writing in my diary, and Sebastian was on Zoom with his uncle Andrew in America. Andrew had planned to come for Elijah's birthday the following week, but no one knew. It made me happy that he had Andrew keeping him company via Zoom. They were playing chess online together. We did not go into surgery until 5:00 pm that evening. We were in the hospital from 11:00 am, and Sebastian had been fasting all day. He was exhausted. I was exhausted. While we were in the pre-admissions area, I texted George and said I could not do this on my own anymore. The COVID rules that were in place that didn't allow patients to have both parents there were incomprehensible.

When they took Sebastian into theatre, I collapsed and started to cry. My wailing echoed throughout the corridor. The emotions of the day had finally caught up with me, and there was no stopping the

Natalie - Life Goes On, But The Tests Do Not Stop

tears that flowed uncontrollably. In the meantime, George spoke to security, informing him of the urgency of being with me. When the nurse walked me out to the waiting area, George stood there as a comforting presence. His hug gave me strength. We made our way to the coffee shop, where we waited for the completion of the surgery. It took one and a half hours, and finally, after what felt like an eternity, we received the call and were told we could see Sebastian. My phone did not stop with calls and messages that day, but I did not have the energy to talk to anyone. George took the calls for me, for which I was truly grateful. George saw Sebastian in recovery, then went home and Sebastian and I went to the ward. The RCH is an exceptional place. We were put in a comfortable private room. Sebastian had a restful night, and then the wait began in the hope that they had removed what was required for the tests. We were discharged the following day at 11:00 am and I drove my brave boy home.

  I had not slept properly in a week. I thought I would go home and crash, but life's business did not allow this to occur. Elijah and Jerome continued school, and it was Elijah's Sports Carnival at a local oval. I felt like we had neglected him all week. I told George I would try to attend, even if only for a short period. Upon arrival, I tried to avoid all the people I knew. Many were unaware of our situation, and I knew that if anyone enquired about my family I would not be able to control my emotions. I approached Elijah, and after embracing him in a hug, he told me he didn't have any lunch. My anger set in. I was angry with George for not realising and with myself for not being on top of things. In hindsight, it

The ~~Worst~~ Best Year

was not a big deal as my youngest child was not the world's greatest eater. However, I was on edge and it did not take much to push me over. I purchased a sausage roll from the bakery up the road and returned with it. As I was leaving the sports ground, I bumped into a friend who asked the dreaded question, "How is the family?" As expected, I broke down. I recall how lovely she was as she comforted me. I pulled myself together and left before anyone else stopped me. That night, I spoke to my boss and informed her I needed indefinite time off work. She was happy for me to work any shift that I could and did not want me to feel under pressure, and I was grateful for this.

Later that week Jerome had his formal. He looked so handsome, and it was just the distraction we needed after the week we had experienced. We had pre-formal drinks at our friend's house; Jerome looked so happy. I was so glad that he was able to be part of this event, as we needed a bit of happiness in our lives right at that moment. Life would continue to move on. People were still celebrating birthdays and weddings. Life did not stop because of what we were experiencing. I wanted to continue to celebrate the events and moments in my eldest and youngest boy's lives despite the ordeal we were experiencing. Their lives were important too.

The next day was Palm Sunday and we all attended church together as a united family. Many of our extended family and friends made an extra effort to attend the same Mass as us. It was a beautiful sunny day. The Palm Sunday Mass was traditionally a children's Mass. It is a Mass that celebrates the children in our Maronite Catholic community.

Natalie - Life Goes On, But The Tests Do Not Stop

Families all come together, and it is one of the happiest occasions in the Church calendar, alongside Christmas. During the Mass, I could not stop crying. I felt so sad. I was trying so hard to stop my tears but to no avail. I was looking around at all the children, and all I could think was, "Why did God choose my son to give this disease to?" I was honestly thinking at the time, "Why choose my child in this church full of children?" This disclosure is the raw and honest truth, and I feel horrible that I even had those thoughts. However, we are all human, and sometimes human emotions are selfish. I think I hid my tears as best as I could that day and made it through Mass.

I had to pull it together for the surprise we had planned for Elijah's birthday. We decided to have Elijah's birthday party five days earlier than his actual birthday and celebrate after the Palm Sunday Mass. Andrew had arrived from the States that morning and was hiding in our guest bedroom. When we all went to church, Andrew and my mother organised everything for the party. When we arrived home, we asked everyone to make their way to the back deck, and we told Elijah that his birthday gift had arrived. Andrew came outside, and everyone was so surprised. It was such a lovely moment. My in-laws were extremely emotional seeing their son was home, even if it was for a short while. It had been two years since they last saw him, so it was an emotional reunion and just what my boys needed. It was the perfect surprise for them and my sister-in-law Gladys, as they were all significantly affected by Sebastian's diagnosis and they all needed a bit of joy to pick them up. Gladys always put her emotions aside to support us in any way she could. Andrew being there was wonderful; now, she had someone to support her. My kids love Uncle Andrew so much and having him with us through those early days was an incredible support to them and the entire family.

Although the afternoon was incredible, celebrating not only Andrew's arrival but Elijah's birthday, I did not sleep at all that night. I knew we were receiving the results in the morning, and that led me to stay up all night worrying. As we were getting ready to leave the following morning, I received a phone call from Dr Claira saying we would have to wait until Wednesday to receive the results, as they had to run more lab tests on the samples. I was devastated as having to wait two more days to find out exactly what we were facing was extremely difficult. I tried to keep it together in front of Sebastian, but I think he could see right through me. He was doing a lot better than I was. My closest friends tried to console me by offering me support, but nothing they said made me feel any better. I had barely made it to Monday, I had to now wait until Wednesday. It was all becoming too much for me. That day was hard on everyone. George and Jerome were very quiet. I could see their minds racing. My friend Monique took Elijah for the day, while my other friend Angela convinced Jerome to hang out with her girls at their house. This all helped, but I could not stop crying. Having the boys out of the house gave me time to myself, so I cried and let all my emotions out.

Tuesday evening, I received a call from Dr Claira asking us to be at the RCH by 9:30 am the next morning. As well as getting his results,

Natalie - Life Goes On, But The Tests Do Not Stop

Sebastian needed to meet with Melbourne IVF. He would need to fast because if they could schedule it, they wanted to surgically insert a port. A port is a device inserted in the chest area to administer chemotherapy. The device is then connected to the veins to allow the chemotherapy to flow through the bloodstream. This was different to my treatment as I received chemotherapy through a cannula inserted into the veins in my hand. A port was usually used when the chemotherapy treatment was going to be long and intense as the port protects the veins. After my last treatment, they could not access my veins and had to swap to the other hand. This would be Sebastian's second surgery in one week.

We arrived at the hospital and met with Dr Claira and another female doctor as Dr Quinn was away. They wasted no time telling us Sebastian had stage four Nodular sclerosis classical Hodgkin lymphoma. It was in his neck, chest, abdomen, groin and bones. It had spread everywhere. I was trying hard to focus on my breathing as I was worried I would collapse in front of him. Luckily, George was allowed to come to this meeting, so I had his support while they explained everything to us. To tell you the truth, I cannot remember what they were saying. It was all white noise. I asked questions but did not even remember the responses, as it was too much to take in. We were expecting it would be advanced, but being told it was stage four hit us for six. How did we go from a perfectly healthy 15-year-old boy to this?

From there, we met with an endocrinologist. Before that day, I had no idea what this type of doctor was. The endocrinologist met with us to talk about freezing Sebastian's sperm. As he was already going through puberty, it was a straightforward procedure, but one I did not want to be a part of. George had already discussed the process with him at home. From day one, I was part of every process he went through, except for this. We drove down to Melbourne IVF, and I went to Lygon St for a coffee while George and Sebastian went to do what needed to be done. He was always such a mature boy. I would never have made him do this if he did not want to. The endocrinologist spoke to him about what was involved. At 15, having children was clearly the furthest thing from his mind, but he thought it best to go through the procedure, just in case.

 After that procedure, we headed back to RCH, hoping that surgery for the port would happen that afternoon. After arriving back, we were told we would instead have to return the next day for the port surgery. One blessing we had was that they did all the preoperative paperwork and the PCR test for COVID-19. This was yet another test I was also stressed about, as Sebastian had been exposed to the virus during the week. COVID was just an added stress to an already highly stressful situation during this time. His PCR was clear, thankfully. Then we received a call from Melbourne IVF saying they needed another sample the following morning. Absolutely nothing was straightforward, and nothing was going to plan. However, in true Sebastian style, he did not complain and agreed to drop off a sample in the morning, as they had requested. They allowed him to do the second sample at home, and we had a 60-minute window to get it to the hospital before it spoiled. These were my potential grand babies swimming in a specimen jar, so

Natalie - Life Goes On, But The Tests Do Not Stop

I told George to put his pedal to the metal and get them to where they needed to be on time. True to form, my champion husband arrived on time with the specimen jar! We joked about it afterwards, saying that if we were pulled over for speeding, we would get the police officers to escort us to Melbourne IVF to get there on time.

When the hospital cancelled the surgery that Wednesday, Sebastian went home to rest from his big day. That night, the Lebanese Church held a Mass dedicated to the sick. Sebastian was too tired to attend so George and I went. I prayed so hard at this Mass. My heart hurt so much, and I kept asking God, "Why is this happening to us?" I just wanted to wake up from this nightmare. I felt like I was running on empty. Two weeks had passed, and I had hardly eaten a single thing. I was getting little to no sleep at all and enduring such long days in the hospital. My weight had dropped to 54 kilograms—a weight I had not been since I was roughly 14. I kept thinking, "If I am feeling like this now, how would I get through the next six to eight months?" At this particular Mass, they gave out Holy Oil which I took home to Sebastian. That healing Mass gave me comfort.

The next morning was April 14. 25 years since George and I had started dating. Who would have thought 25 years prior that our lives would have taken us down the paths it had? Again, I did not sleep that night. I was reflecting on my beautiful family. I was reflecting on the beautiful relationship that George and I had. A lot had happened in those years. When I was diagnosed with cancer, my relationship with George strengthened. He supported me in every way. He made me feel beautiful when I felt so ugly, but during that time, I was not the angry person that I had become now. When I was sick I never asked, "Why me?" This time every day I woke up and asked, "Why Sebastian?" When I was sick, I was scared, not angry. I was scared that if I died, who would look after my children? However, George always made me feel secure. Now I was always angry, an anger like I had never felt before. I was sad, a sadness that I could not even explain. I was scared, like having a nightmare which you can't wake up from. That day, I prayed that our love, the love we had nurtured over 25 years, would conquer all these emotions. Thank God it did. Again, it made us even stronger. It was not always 'love songs and dedications', but we worked through the hard times to make our relationship stronger. There were many times when I was staying in the hospital with Sebastian, and George was at home looking after the boys, that I would call him and take out my frustrations on him. He never held anything I said against me.

We arrived at the hospital in the morning and were informed it was going to be an early afternoon surgery. George was working out of his car to be close to us in case I needed him. Again, COVID did not allow him (as the second parent) to come into the hospital to offer us support. Emergency patients delayed the surgery, so I sent George home. There was no point in him waiting in the car all day. I hoped the surgery would happen early so we could return home, as the next day was Good Friday and Elijah's 11th birthday. All the waiting was making Sebastian very frustrated. *Peppa Pig* playing on the hospital TV was not helping one bit. It was playing all day. Sebastian was hungry, tired and looked stressed. He snapped back every time I looked in his direction. I spoke to the nurse at 2:00 pm, and she told us to go for a walk and that they would call us when they were ready. I was stressed because I was worried that we would wait all this time only to be sent home again. Half an hour later, we received the call to come back up. He finally went in for surgery at 3:30 pm. The surgeon informed me that the surgery should take around one and a half hours, and after he came out of recovery, he could return home. I kissed him as he went under, and again, I fell apart. Walking out of Admissions on my own, I was completely broken. I received a message from my old high school friend saying she was coming in to wait with me. Seeing her waiting for me downstairs was just what I needed. She gave me a big hug while I cried. I can't even explain the loneliness of it all. People would ask, "What can we do?" It is not something you could verbalise, but there were gestures like holding me while I cried that gave me comfort. I was grateful that Marianna was there, and she waited with me until the surgery was over.

 Thankfully, the surgery went well, and they decided as it was so late, they would keep Sebastian overnight and begin chemotherapy in the morning. We were so lucky that we celebrated Elijah's birthday earlier, as we would spend his actual birthday in the hospital.

Chapter 8

Are We Really Talking Fertility?

~ *Sebastian* ~

Within one week of my initial scan, I had a confirmed diagnosis of stage IV cancer, a port inserted into me, and I had started chemotherapy. Alongside the multitude of burdens associated with receiving chemotherapy was the potential for a loss in fertility. We had an appointment booked with the endocrinologist at the RCH. Unlike oncologists, who have a special understanding of cancer, endocrinologists have a specialised understanding of cell signalling, including hormones. The appointment with them was to determine my stage of puberty and a plan for managing the risk to my fertility during chemo. For some reason, we would be seeing the endocrinologists from the cancer ward instead of a specific part of the hospital. I wasn't sure why, maybe something to do with all the cancer children needing endocrinology support, but I wasn't complaining because it was easier for me. Despite being there to see the endocrinologist, I couldn't escape the depressing waiting room of

Sebastian - Are We Really Talking Fertility?

the specialist Clinic E at the RCH, reserved for cancer treatment. Again, I was conscious of the contrast between the colour of the paintings, the flyers around me, and the sickness of the children. Some were happy, others didn't care or didn't really know what their cancer meant, some didn't want to be there, and some were just flat-out in pain. No one seemed to be in a complete state of happiness when waiting.

"Sebastian!" I was up, and the wait time was actually not too bad, which was pleasing. It was an early morning session so that's probably why. The doctor explained how chemo affects fertility significantly, and I had a four in five chance of my fertility being very damaged, given the high intensity of chemo that I would be receiving. She said she needed to take measurements of the reproductive organs to determine how progressed I was into puberty and what options I had. My parents left the room, and the measurements were taken. It was really awkward and felt unnecessary, but if it meant saving my ability to have children, then I was all for it. The doctor noted that I was "developed" enough through puberty. Basically, I had two options: do nothing, but as I was likely to be infertile, I would have no chance of having children, or alternatively, I could store some sperm in the interim before treatment and use it down the track if I was infertile after treatment. There was no real downside to submitting a sample as it would be stored for free until I turned 18. By then, I would be able to find out if I was fertile and make a choice about it. So it was a no-brainer and we had to take a drive to the andrology clinic, where I would submit a sample.

The drive over was very awkward but luckily not too long. We had to be back at the hospital later that day for another appointment, so there was time to kill anyway, which made this trip well-timed. The car ride was quite silent as we approached the clinic. Worse yet, there were not many parking spots available, so we were left circling the same street until a spot opened up for us. This was not very favourable given we had to be back at the hospital as soon as we could to make our next appointment. Walking into the front door of the clinic was very sketchy. The building from the outside seemed old, and there were two locked doors, separated by a small space, to enter the building. There was also one of those signs remnant of COVID telling you to wear a mask. We had to press a buzzer to get someone's attention, and even that looked outdated. The inside carpet was worse for wear, and the interior dimly lit. Then my dad took it upon himself to ask whether I knew how to, you know, submit the sample. As if the day could not get any more awkward.

    Thankfully, we were the only ones around, so there was no wait. I was given a clipboard to fill out with my details. The boxes were your typical name, address, phone number, the works. Now it was time. I would be left alone in the bathroom to do my business and while I'll have to spare you most of the details, I think you can imagine the discomfort of doing it in a urine sample cup on the toilet. Anyway, leaving the andrology clinic was a relief to say the least. On the way out, I caught a glimpse of the lab room with all their equipment, and I couldn't help but hold onto the mental image of them counting my sperm as soon as I left them. It was back to hospital time, and I was glad to be on my way.

The drive over was filled with twists and turns past Melbourne University buildings. It can be hard during times like these, when there appears to be a lot of really important things going on with your life, to remember where you're heading and what your future holds. Part of being in survival mode is living in the present. Sure, I did all that I needed to keep future options open, I am not silly, but I often didn't give my future as much thought. Instead, I preferred to focus on my treatment and survival. It was about time for lunch, so as soon as we finished up at the hospital, we found the nearest cafe to grab a bite.

The cafes at the hospital were your typical overpriced, run-of-the-mill places. There weren't many options, but Mum would often use her free coffee vouchers from one particular cafe when she had some time on her hands. One of the charity organisations was able to get her a 10 free coffee voucher to use when I was receiving treatment, so we often ate there or at the very least, Mum did, and I got food from somewhere else. Most of what the cafes offered were wraps and rolls so I would find myself time and time again trying a new mix of ingredients between two pieces of bread. The cafes were also a chance to relax after a stressful day. The feeling that you get when you sit or lie down after working hard physically or mentally is exceedingly liberating. The freedom from labour and intense thought is underrated. Being someone who likes to, and often is, forced to push themselves, I am blessed with this feeling quite often but it never gets old. Furthermore, it's hard to feel too guilty about sitting down and taking a break after you have been working hard. Today, my work wasn't too difficult, but I had recently had some difficult things thrown at me, and the awkwardness about literally everything happening on this particular day could make anyone feel lucky that it was over. Or well, so one might think.

"Sebastian, the andrologists just called."

"Already! That was fast. What did they say?"

"They said that your sperm is reasonably viable but they don't have enough to fill the desired amount of vials, so they are going to need you to submit another sample."

Seriously? I was just liberated from all this stuff and now they wanted me to come back? I didn't have to worry about it just at that moment, but I was going to have to worry about it sooner or later.

"They said you can do it from home this time as long as you drop off the sample within the hour."

Well at least it wouldn't be so weird this time and it wouldn't be as disgusting as the stool test, plus we wouldn't have to be waiting around until I had to go, so I guess it wasn't the worst thing in the world. Surely enough, I did what I had to do the next morning, bagged and passed off the vial to my dad to deliver to their doorstep. Thank goodness that was over. The thing that annoys me the most is that I am going to have to do it all again when I choose to retest my fertility down the track, which ought to be fun. Until that day, we can joke about my lack of fertility since I am unlikely to have the fastest of swimmers left. Ever since I started treatment, any time I was close to being hit or hurt in that area, the go-to joke has been for Mum to remind us that she wants grandkids, and for us to tell her that I probably won't be giving her any by natural means anyway. So it doesn't matter how hard I'm hit, so long as I am still in one piece.

Chapter 9

The First Day Of Chemo

~ *Sebastian* ~

It's Good Friday 2022. The bustling atmosphere of the RCH is indubitably evident amidst the campaigning of the Good Friday Appeal. If you are unaware, the Good Friday Appeal is a well-known public fundraising event in Australia where people around the state of Victoria donate to support Melbourne's RCH. The total donations for the event had been increasing exponentially over the passing decades and this year appeared to be no exception. There were rides to enjoy, a media crew present, and scores of famous people including (but not limited to) professional footballers from around the state. Visitor restrictions were relaxed for the day to allow families to celebrate the fundraising festivities with their loved ones.

 Despite the many activities on display at the hospital, the more exigent matter at hand was receiving life-saving cancer treatment. Within the previous 12 hours, I had just completed surgery to implant a

Sebastian - The First Day of Chemo

port for ease of chemotherapy treatment. The port was only visible as a small, round bump on the side of my chest and thus, for the most part, I wouldn't even notice its presence unless I was physically looking at it. It could cause some issues when it came to trying to go to sleep with the port accessed (i.e. it had the needle still in). Whenever accessed, I was constantly worrying about accidentally rolling over on it in my sleep and hurting myself, so I made sure to sleep on my opposite side, and I sometimes even adjusted my pillow to provide the needle some support so I didn't push it into me.

The oncologists assigned to my treatment, along with the other staff at the hospital, were keen for me to begin treatment. I found myself in the Kelpie Ward of the hospital, dedicated to adolescents and people undergoing cancer treatment. Each ward of the hospital had a very Australian name with most being named after native Australian wildlife. In my hospital room I had the basics: a bed to sleep in, a bedside table, a TV, and a multitude of medical equipment. Periodically, nurses would check in on me and see how I was recovering from the surgery whilst informing me about what I would need to prepare for regarding my chemotherapy treatment. The surgery had left me with a burning sensation in my mouth from the breathing tube that the doctors used to assist them in the operating room. Unfortunately for me, this meant that I had an annoying pain in my throat, as if I had a bad cold, for the next one to two days.

"Do you want some pain medication for your throat?" asked the nurse. Thinking that some pain relief wouldn't be such a bad idea, I agreed to have Tramadol, an opioid, to overcome the pain despite not having had it before. Because I was about to begin chemo, I wasn't allowed to receive ibuprofen as it is an anti-inflammatory medication that could enhance the unwanted effects of chemo. As the chemo kills rapidly dividing cells, your blood count often takes an Olympic dive during treatment, and further hampering inflammatory and clotting abilities during treatment is strongly advised against. For me, this meant avoiding ibuprofen medications such as Nurofen and trying others such as Tramadol to manage the pain, although it probably wasn't the best idea to add another medication that was known to induce nausea on my first day of chemo.

Before I could begin treatment, my port (the device used to administer chemo) needed to be accessed. This involved a long, fine needle shaped like an 'L' being injected into the site where I had received surgery just hours prior, and securing the needle with a range of bandages and support. To mitigate the pain, a numbing cream was used. The nurse looking after me on that day was Rickey. I would often have Rickey as one of my oncology nurses. He was one of many we would get to know well over my journey. He was a pretty interesting and laid-back person. There weren't many male nurses in the hospital, so to have Rickey around was nice. The coolness of the cream felt relieving on my burning, scarred skin. It was like using a block of ice to anaesthetise my wound. For the numbing cream to be effective, it needed to be applied for at least half an hour prior to treatment. Hence, I still had 30 minutes before I would begin my very first session of chemo.

Sebastian - The First Day of Chemo

My anticipation was now building from within. Nervous and excited, I patiently awaited the all-clear from the medical staff and the beginning of my treatment. There was ample coverage of the Good Friday Appeal on TV, so of course given that I was staying at the RCH, it was only fitting that I watched it. It never really dawned on me that I had missed a lot of church that week. I had been brought up in a Catholic household so Holy Week (Palm Sunday to Easter Sunday) often involved a lot of going to church. However, as I was so invested in focusing on my treatment, I did not give much thought to the fact that I was missing it.

The idea of faith during treatment varies tremendously from person to person. My faith didn't change much throughout my journey. Having such high confidence in those around me was all I needed to surmount the emotional affliction that is attached to such a traumatic experience. Whilst I have had an affinity for science for many years, as I emerged from life with cancer, I noticed that I became more and more obsessed with the health sciences and everything tangible. Biology was my favourite subject in the year that followed, and I would do many practice biology exams for the fun of learning. So maybe I didn't change spiritually over the cancer journey, but I felt as though my connections to health and science were stronger than ever. I didn't think the same could be said for my mother. Instead, she seemed to ride the ups and downs of faith during my treatment, which makes sense given what was happening at the time.

After a while of waiting, the doctors entered my room and the confidence in their strut told me that it was time. I was about to start my

The ~~Worst~~ Best Year

first session of chemotherapy. The chemo treatment involved the use of a machine that would transport chemicals to the port so that they could be intravenously pushed around my body. On this day, I would go on to receive four different chemo drugs, one of which, prednisolone, was a steroid. The other three were doxorubicin, vincristine, and etoposide. Each drug had specific side effects, however the one point of similarity between them all, apart from their ability to treat cancer, was that one way or another they made me feel sick. There were four hours of chemo to enjoy that day, so I decided to make myself comfortable. Piled under several thin white hospital sheets and crawled up on the side of the bed, I gave myself some time to relax.

  This didn't last long though, as I was greeted by the screams and interruptions of my family. Understandably, my parents were fussing over every little detail down to the lighting in the room, but my little brother could not be any happier among the many football players there for the Good Friday celebrations, many of whom played for Carlton (the team our family supports). There was a lot of waiting around during chemo given how long it lasted—and half that time was spent waiting to start. I knew my mum wanted to take lots of photos to capture the experience but seemed a little reluctant. She told me that she would only take what I allowed her to. I also wanted to save the memories, so I instructed her at every corner to do so. There were plenty of photos to be taken on days like today, milestones of progressing in treatment, where the family could gather around together.

  After the chemo finally began, Dad took my little brother Elijah

Sebastian - The First Day of Chemo

to explore the hospital and all the events that were on at the time. Football players, musicians, and more, there was plenty to keep them occupied. Lucky for Elijah, as it was his birthday, getting to run around the hospital and meet all of his favourite national celebrities was an amazing gift for him, especially because he was 11 years old and sports-obsessed. I figured it would be best to find something to keep me busy, and I naturally found myself watching some YouTube. Since it was still school holidays, I didn't have much homework, so I enjoyed watching TV and YouTube as much as I wanted at this point.

The only problem was that every half an hour or so, I would be interrupted by the beeping of the IV machine. The machine would go off whenever it finished a chemo cycle, flushing out a cycle with saline, whenever it was low on battery, whenever it had become stuck, or whenever it felt like annoying me. Therefore, I soon became accustomed to the silence button while waiting for a nurse to come and take care of the machine. In between the machine beeping, waiting for the nurse, getting hooked up to a new drug, and watching YouTube, I was able to speak to Carlton footballer Ed Curnow, whom Elijah and Dad had run into on the ground floor. Since players were not allowed into the hospital wards and rooms due to COVID-19 restrictions on visitors, I received the second best and met with Curnow online, COVID style. Along with the FaceTime call came signed Carlton gear, memorable enough to brighten an already interesting day.

Before I knew it, the etoposide was completed and next was the doxorubicin, aka 'the red devil'. The drug is commonly referred to by this name, given its distinct and vibrant red colour. It was known to turn bodily fluids such as urine, but also tears, red and was infamous for causing severe sickness amongst those who received it. No longer was I very nervous. Now, raging pure excitement was all I could feel; I wanted to know what it would be like to receive the drug. I wanted to know whether I would cry or pee red. Unfortunately, for me, I didn't cry close to receiving the drug and so I didn't get the opportunity to expel tears the colour of blood. However, I did get to pee and the tinge of red in my urine this time and every time I urinated after receiving this drug were the highlights of my days. I know it sounds weird and nerdy, but I was genuinely excited to see my urine turn red. It's not every day that you look down in the toilet and see red instead of the usual yellow, at least not for me. The doxorubicin was administered with a slightly different IV machine. I never really asked about or remembered asking why, although maybe it had something to do with its potency or packaging.

    To change me from etoposide to doxorubicin, Rickey had to unplug one of the three wires coming out from my port, place the syringe holding the doxorubicin into the new IV machine, and re-hook me into that one. In contrast to the traditional chemo machine which emptied the chemical from a plastic bag through a tube that ran into my port, this machine would slowly push what was essentially a syringe filled with 30mLs of the chemical into a line that connected to my port. This machine was a bit scarier. Its exterior was darker, and it made more sounds than the other machine, not to mention that its silence button

Sebastian - The First Day of Chemo

was in a different place and it took me a while to find it. Even after I located it, the machine would only stay quiet for about a minute until it would start beeping again and I would have to re-silence it. As the nurses were very busy, it would often take them a good five minutes to come and take care of the machine. However, before the nurses could come, I needed to also press the nurse-call button, an elliptic green button located at the bottom of the TV remote. After looking around for a bit to find it, I felt a little anxious pressing it. I hadn't pressed the button in recent memory and wasn't sure whether I was even supposed to call a nurse over something like this. Nevertheless, I pressed the button. I would be left silencing the machine, waiting, and then silencing again several times per drug and flush cycle until the nurse arrived.

As it was the Good Friday Appeal, there was also an endless supply of merchandise on offer to purchase. My little brother opted to take full advantage of this and purchased an RCH t-shirt. It was one of those 'I heart x' t-shirts with x of course being RCH. In addition to the t-shirt was an RCH-themed Monopoly. This was a superb way to pass some time on those long days when I was pinned to the hospital bed and the confines of my room. When Dad and Elijah returned to the chemo room, we thought it best to bust out the Monopoly to pass the time. "Do you want us to bring it to you?" Mum asked. It made the most sense, rather than having to unplug 5000 cords attached to my machine and carry it around with me. The whole family jumped on different parts of the bed with the bedside table making an excellent base to put the Monopoly on. I could tell you how the game went, although we would be here for a little while, not to mention we never finished it because of all the interruptions throughout the day.

Three times a day, I would take a dosage of 32.5 milligrams of prednisolone. It is quite crazy to think about how I was having just shy of 0.1 grams of the steroids, and about 100mLs of every drug combined, yet they had such strong and lasting impacts on me and took so long to be administered. After receiving the doxorubicin, I was just left with a short dosage of 25 mLs of vincristine. This ran over as little as 15 minutes with five additional minutes to flush the remaining chemotherapy out of the line running into my port. Overall, I didn't mind how this was much shorter than the hour each for doxorubicin and etoposide with 17-minute flushes. Some people wonder whether you can feel the chemo coming into your body, however, the short answer is no. Since the chemo that I was receiving was pushed through the body at such a slow rate, it is hard to notice it. The main struggle of receiving chemo, apart from the time and effort it takes for it to be administered, is the aftermath at home when you become sick as a result of receiving the treatment. Despite this, when large quantities of saline are pushed through a syringe, particularly if the syringe was connected to my arm instead of my port, I could feel it. The rush of coolness would be exhilarating on the skin. It felt as though the site of the syringe was leaking, but in actual fact, it was purely a sensation from the saline being pushed through.

The end of chemo was an entire process. On the days that I had another session of chemo scheduled for the following day, I would keep

Sebastian - The First Day of Chemo

my port accessed overnight. To do this, however, Rickey still had to pump the anticoagulant heparin into my port to prevent clots overnight while it was still accessed. The process was simple as the needle would be staying in. Rickey gloved up and unclipped all lines that connected me to the IV machine. He then pushed saline through my line and a small dose of heparin, and I was good to go. My mum and dad were not sure as to whether I would be okay to walk to the car, but I thought I'd be fine so I walked down to the car park without help. Thinking I had gotten past the panicking obsession over every detail from my parents would be a mistake because I think they told me that I was walking too fast half a dozen times on the way down, and that I should take things "slowly, slowly". Any slower and I would have been going backwards.

Upon completion of my first chemo, my uncle George called asking if he could come over to visit along with my aunt Gladys. As I am always keen to see visitors, I approved. But I had barely anticipated the obvious effects that the chemo would have on me in the short term. Soon after walking through the door at home, I had the urgent sensation that told me I needed to expel everything in my stomach one way or another. In no more than a second, I was off to the bathroom, walking at first and then bolting like it was the 100-metre sprint on athletics day. I just made it in time. Unfazed, I returned to the living room as if it were any other day and tried to act 'normal'. Part of the issue was that I was running on no antiemetic medication at the time to prevent nausea and sickness so it was not long before I was bolting to the bathroom again. This time we were prepared and had a bucket on site in addition to my vomit bag, which I tried to avoid using if I could make it to the bathroom. Again, unfazed I continued to act as if everything was normal, but Mum and Dad understandably wanted me to rest.

I have spent my whole life trying to be unique and enjoy everything, good or bad, that made me different. Going upstairs it was as if what was happening to me had started to hit me. I was not normal anymore, no matter how hard I tried to be at such an abnormal time. I threw up another two times that night, each less impressive than the last with less in my body to expel as time went on. From that point on, I barely spent a single moment whilst receiving chemo without ample antiemetics to calm the risk of vomiting. These worked extremely well, and I only actually puked one more time throughout the rest of my treatment. Moreover, on the one occasion where I did throw up, I hadn't had my dosage of anti-nausea medication. Whilst the meds didn't circumvent the range of events where I was feeling quite sick, I never threw up when receiving the flurry of anti-nausea medication prescribed. These medications included ondansetron, cyclizine, fosaprepitant, and lorazepam. The four medications, in particular fosaprepitant and ondansetron, would manage to save me on numerous occasions from the burdens of sickness posed by the chemotherapy medications.

I laid down in bed that night, beginning to adjust to a 'lazy lifestyle' where I was starting to focus on relaxing with a bit of schoolwork rather than working with a bit of relaxation. As it was school holidays, I didn't actually do schoolwork for a few weeks, however, when school came back, I ended up spending a lot less time studying than I was used to.

Sebastian - The First Day of Chemo

This was a massive challenge for me mentally given my absurd obsession with working hard and being productive. More than a year later, looking back on my experience, I wish I had completed more homework during my sickness. One thing to learn from my experience with cancer was just like during COVID lockdowns, it can be easy to adjust to a new routine once you are in it. It feels standard to you, you barely notice how different your workload was to a year prior. While this may have worked against me during treatment, I still made sure I worked hard enough to reasonably maintain my stellar grades at school. Part of me wonders whether I just felt like I was less productive because I managed to find a way to cut out all of the unnecessary parts of Year 10 whilst focusing my time on the important ones. This made it seem like I was working less when in actual fact, I was being just as productive. Nevertheless, after chemo I quickly adjusted to a large workload, which was not too hard to maintain once I became used to it.

Chapter 10

Cancer Didn't Make Us Sick, Chemo Did

~ *Natalie* ~

Cancer is a force that defies logic and reason. I can think of many words to describe cancer, but both Sebastian and I did not look sick. For me, it was an itchy scalp and a lump in my neck. For Sebastian, it was a crazy, intense itch all over his body and unusual blood results, but we did not look sick. There was no way that Sebastian looked like he had cancer, let alone stage four. Looking sick began with the treatment. This poison that they pump into our bodies ultimately saved our lives but made us so sick. It is so toxic that if it touches your skin, it could cause burns so severe that you would require skin grafts. Body fluids should not be exchanged for 48 hours after treatment. This poison is so toxic that it is recommended that other family members use a different toilet to the one you use, or if you are sharing a toilet, you need to full flush and use the toilet cleaner immediately afterwards. Chemotherapy is so toxic that when you vomit, you need to ensure that you do not handle the cleaning up of the contents you've expelled with your bare hands; you are encouraged to wear gloves. However, it is this toxic medication that saved our lives.

I know when I was receiving chemotherapy treatment, there were many times that I refused to look at myself in the mirror. This may sound vain, but many people have always complimented my hair. It was something that little girls at my children's school would comment on. Strangers would stop me to say you have the most beautiful hair. I remember when I was dating George, he would always compliment me on my hair. Over the years my weight would fluctuate up and down and I wasn't always comfortable, but my hair was a different story entirely. My hair was always something that I was happy with, and when it began to fall out, I was devastated. I gained a lot of weight and did not look pale; I looked grey. My nails were extremely brittle and had started to turn purple. When my nail colour began to change I had a panic attack, but was reassured by a friend who had experienced the same thing that it was very normal. Some people lose their nails; luckily, Sebastian and I didn't. Sebastian and I were so constipated most of the time. My period stopped, and there was a chance that early menopause would occur but my period returned after treatment. The funny thing was I went into menopause when Sebastian was diagnosed. My period was due the week he was diagnosed, and it never returned since that time. My doctor said that I was put into stress-induced menopause. I had the worst heartburn going through treatment, and so did Sebastian. My heartburn was more like a stomach burn. I was so uncomfortable all the time. After my radiation, I suffered from a severe dry mouth for years. My teeth became so sensitive that even the cold wind made them hurt. The dry mouth at night really bothered me, and currently does, and it wakes me up on most nights. Almost ten years on, the symptoms have lingered. It took years for my energy levels to return to normal.

My symptoms were nothing compared to what Sebastian went through. It was heartbreaking to see how sick he was. My beautiful boy faced every obstacle thrown at him like a champion. He told many jokes throughout his ordeal and continued to smile his way through the entire experience. I even felt that he supported us through his sickness. Many times, he would withhold the pain he was experiencing or push aside the nausea that lingered so as not to worry me. I went through chemotherapy, but there was no comparison to the intensity of his treatment plan. He would require treatment for 15 days and then rest for 15 days before it would begin all over again. Rounds one and two were tough, with four-to-five-hour days, but when we started rounds three to six, that chemotherapy regime was gruelling. The first two days of each round were long. Some days, he was hooked up for eight to nine hours, and then we would return to the hospital the next day to do it all again. We would leave the hospital at 6:00 pm to return the following day at 8:00 am. He never complained or gave up. He did what needed to be done, while I was the one who cried myself to sleep, wanting to give up. My son was so sick, isolated from friends and family, and not once did he complain. Watching him through this experience was almost too much for me to bear.

Natalie - Cancer Didn't Make Us Sick, Chemo Did

With every round of chemotherapy, we ended up in the emergency department for some reason or another. Many times we ended up in hospital for an illness, and Sebastian would have to be given IV antibiotics. Then there was a time when the pain in his legs was so bad that he could not walk. The steroids were killing his bones, and this was a massive problem as the steroids were part of the chemotherapy treatment and stopping them was not an option that they wanted to consider. I can recall hearing him moaning into his pillow from pain so that no one would hear him because that was the kind of child he was. He did not want to worry us.

There were also many blood transfusions, and this was something I struggled with. The first time they told us he needed a blood transfusion, I felt sick to my stomach. He had been through so much already, and the idea of giving him someone else's blood didn't sit well with me. George gives blood every 90 days. I have always approved of this and thought it was a wonderful gift he was giving. I never really understood how blood transfusions worked. There was a whole process involved before the blood was administered. Lots of tests needed to happen, and we had to wait, hoping his haemoglobin levels would increase. When they don't improve on their own, then a blood transfusion is required. I wanted them to take a family member's blood, but the doctors refused. They explained that the blood goes through many stages before being given to a patient. After many discussions with the doctors, we agreed.

The first time he was given blood it had to be administered very slowly, and the nurse needed to stay by his bed for almost the whole

The ~~Worst~~ Best Year

time as his body could reject the blood, and he could have an allergic reaction as a result. Every time the nurse left the room, she would tell me to keep an eye on him, and she would return promptly. We developed a rapport with this particular nurse, and there was a lot of banter over tennis as we watched Wimbledon. She told Sebastian that she did not like Nick Kyrgios, and he would joke about Nick not needing her approval. Sebastian would talk to her about his strengths and skills as a tennis player. They spent the whole time joking about Nick Kyrgios, and it was a nice distraction from the vampire vibes I was feeling as I watched the blood drip into my son's body. He received the blood well, his blood count increased, and I thought it was over. However, with every chemotherapy round, we ended up back in the Emergency Department to receive more blood or to be put on an IV to receive antibiotics, and sometimes it was to get both at the same time.

When you are receiving chemotherapy, you must take your temperature daily. If your temperature hits 38°C, you must go to the hospital emergency department. With Sebastian, his smartwatch would usually let us know when it was time to go to the hospital, as his heart rate would become so high that his watch would alert him that something was wrong. His heart rate would increase before the temperature rise would kick in. By the time we arrived at the hospital, his temperature would have hit 40. In the six months that Sebastian went through treatment, we spent more time in the hospital than we did at home.

So many times you hear about the wait times at the Children's

Natalie - Cancer Didn't Make Us Sick, Chemo Did

Hospital. These wait times are so long that it even makes it to the news. Even in the days of COVID, when they were severely understaffed, we never waited. Every time we arrived at the Emergency Department, we were taken straight in and put into a private cubicle. Sebastian's blood count was low which meant he could not be exposed to other patients as this would cause a risk of infections. One night there was no room for us, so they treated us in what looked like a storeroom. It was a room with a couch, stored Christmas ornaments, and a cabinet stocked with muesli bars, and we sat in that room for hours. The nurses would come in, check on him, and apologise. They felt bad, but we loved being there. They were still caring for him, and we were far away from the sadness and sickness that enveloped the Emergency Department.

We had the best night together, joking and playing *Bananagrams*, a word game that we loved to play on every hospital trip. Sebastian FaceTimed Martine and Julian, his mates who he calls his cousins, and they stayed on the phone with him for hours keeping him company. Although I knew he was very unwell that night, it was so nice to see him joking and laughing with his friends. They wanted him to open a box of muesli bars to see what they tasted like. He did, and it was an ongoing joke that continued between them. It was Martine's birthday just after that trip, so we took her a box of muesli bars and added them to her birthday gift as a joke.

Chapter 11

My Bones Are Dying

~ *Sebastian* ~

Imagine the sharpest pain you have ever felt. Excruciating, nightmarish, suffering, my bones were dying, and my legs were temporarily made redundant as I struggled to move them. I spent a large portion of my time when undergoing chemo attempting to run from the pain and discomfort associated with it. On the 12th day of my first treatment cycle, I was struck with agony in my lower body. I looked over at my phone, but even that was too much effort. "Hey Google, call Mum." The ringing of all the other Google devices in the house was loud enough to hear from my room, but such ringing never stopped. There was no answer, but not because no one cared to answer. I immediately heard thumping on the staircase, the rattling of our metal handrail on the stairs and screams of confusion as pandemonium erupted in the Khoury household. I heard, "What happened? Did someone hurt themselves?" It turned out that rather than take the time to answer the

Sebastian - My Bones Are Dying

Google device, my parents thought it would be wiser to rush up the staircase and come straight to me.

I explained the pain to them, and they gave me paracetamol for some relief (I was still unable to take ibuprofen or any anti-inflammatory medication at the time as that could exacerbate the adverse effects of chemo on my blood counts). Minutes passed, then ten, then twenty. Whilst the paracetamol had time to start taking effect, the pain was only intensifying. Either I had just had two very large Tic Tacs or this thing was no joke. For the first time throughout this experience and maybe even ever, I was experiencing excruciating pain, a consistent nine out of ten. The pain was felt from my hips to my shins and everywhere in between. Sticking it through the severe pain was twice the challenge as enduring the constant nausea I grappled with at the start of chemo. It wasn't until I was given oxycodone that it settled.

As someone who seeks out logic and reasoning in their life, I aim to only trust certain sources of information that have been supported by extensive evidence. In contrast, my parents are stronger advocates for holistic approaches to treatments. This gives rise to many arguments, as my parents try to convince me of the benefits of their herbal approaches, which I see no value in. I'm not by any means trying to portray my parents negatively because they didn't deny the benefits of a more 'scientific' approach to treatment, but they also wanted me to try and incorporate alternate methods as well. To cut a long story short, they would go on to request that I see a herbal specialist for the pain in my legs, and me having better things to do, would deny such requests.

The ~~Worst~~ Best Year

Less than a week later, the pain was back, awakening me from my sleep without a care in the world. If it was going to ruin my day by putting me in agony, the least my legs could do was wait until a reasonable hour. No one was up as it was still in the early hours of the morning. No one was around to help. Worse yet, the burning in my legs showed no signs of slowing down. I was going to have to do something or brave the pain. I used my hand to feel around my bedhead for the medications, to no avail. After our last trip to the hospital, we were given a prescription for oxycodone to manage the leg pain should it arise again. But the oxycodone was only helpful if I could get to it. After laying in bed, enduring the relentless sharpness in my legs, I decided to go downstairs and try to find the medication.

I leant up with my upper body, the part of me that still worked. Then slowly but surely, I lifted my sheets off me and using my hands, turned my legs to face the side of my bed. Then one foot at a time, I made my way downstairs. The pain was only worsening with my movement and in between each step, I wondered whether my bones would break if I landed forcefully on my next step. Meanwhile, I was shaking profusely, rattling the handrail that took me downstairs. Hopefully, I wasn't about to wake someone up. I briefly looked around for the medicine but couldn't see it. The drugs were not going to be worth the effort of searching around for them. Back to bed it was so I could spend the next few hours tossing and turning in pain.

After spending most of the last few weeks at home, my parents thought it would be beneficial if I returned to school. In fact, Mum and

Sebastian - My Bones Are Dying

Dad strongly suggested that I need to get back into the classroom (oblivious to knowing the extent of my pain at the time because I didn't want to worry them). As my parents seemed keen on me going, I thought, *why not?* As I approached the gates of my high school, I was excited, a weird emotion for a teenager approaching school for sure. However, after spending a little while away from it, coming back felt important and right. Maybe it would be a way to boost productivity, but at the very least, it would give me some opportunity to see my friends.

I moved through the school gates, past the big welcoming school sign and headed to my locker. However, my legs refused to move faster than a snail's pace. I took one slow step at a time, holding onto the shaking rail for dear life. I made my way down the stairs slowly enough to ensure my legs wouldn't give out from under me. I could feel the heat of everyone's eyes burning into me. I was the centre of attention. As I approached my locker and bent over to open it, I realised my legs were not sturdy enough to carry me if I bent my knees. I chose to sit on the ground in a very awkward position that allowed me to open the locker. I put my bag in, and slowly, one step at a time yet again, I moved at a snail's pace back up the stairs to class, where my double period of biochemistry awaited me. The problem was that the classroom was halfway across the school and up four flights of stairs. To my right, boys scaled the staircase, skipping every second step and flying through the corridors. What took me a near minute, these boys had achieved in a matter of seconds. Walking around the school like an injured penguin was bound to raise a few eyebrows, and that it did! My year-level coordinator took note and tried checking in on me. I shrugged such comments off because I figured I would best handle things on my own, even if it took me longer to get to my class.

As expected, everyone who saw me was curious about where I had been, so I told them the truth. They were visibly shocked, and not many knew how to respond. They tried to be as supportive yet apologetic as possible, and it helped to make me feel supported. I had told my close friends, who already knew about my diagnosis, to not tell anyone else because I wanted to be the one to tell the first few people from my school. Everyone else who ever knew me proceeded to find out soon after, as news of my diagnosis entrenched itself within every social network I was directly and indirectly connected to. People I hadn't seen for years soon found out and got in contact with me to check in. They even sent gifts, including a thoughtful package from someone I hadn't seen since primary school. The world now knew about me, and there was no stopping the doughnut deliveries that followed.

Entering the classroom, I immediately sensed that things were right and that I was back where I belonged. I could feel the joy around me as people who I hadn't seen for weeks were back in the same room as me. These emotions were short-lived as they were dampened by the throbbing pain in my hips. It was literally like the bones within me were dying, and I was helpless to conquer it. Despite this, I urged myself to mask it, to appear strong in this time of weakness. I would focus on learning and science for the moment. When I was learning, I was in control and able to block out the horrors of everything else in my life.

Sebastian - My Bones Are Dying

While I was able to turn a blind eye to these horrors, not everyone did. When I arrived home, my mum informed me that my year-level coordinator had called and told her that he saw me walking a little funny and wanted to make sure that I was okay. Honestly, I wasn't and the longer it took to find the source of my pain, the longer it would be before I could resolve it.

We of course raised this concern with the doctors, and they were unsure about the cause. Briefly, the idea of me having avascular necrosis was raised, however, to be diagnosed with this condition usually required a person to have used an excessive amount of steroids and/or alcohol over a multi-year period. Since I had only received 12 days of chemo at the time, it was highly unlikely. It was essentially unheard of for someone to develop such an ailment. We considered getting an MRI to understand what was happening, but since the pain only lasted a few hours at a time, we opted to put the MRI on hold for a while longer.

Within a matter of days, the pain I found myself in led me to make an unscheduled trip to the hospital. It was always hard to tell what level of illness constituted a trip there, but sometimes it is important to trust your gut. This would become one of many unscheduled trips I would make to the RCH. Coming out of the elevator, I was confronted by the COVID-19 check-in desk with a typical line of people waiting in four lanes. Each lane had at least a dozen people. I had no patience to stand and wait in long lines for extensive periods. Just then, a security guard rushed towards us, pushing a wheelchair. Having noticed my pain, he helped us, and we bypassed the COVID queues. My parents snapped

The ~~Worst~~ Best Year

up this opportunity faster than the receptionist could scribble my name down on a post-it note for COVID prevention purposes and slap it on my jumper. I felt a sense of importance while I was rushed past the sea of people standing in the queue at the check-in area. At this moment, I could fully admire the ability of hospitals to prioritise patients not by race, wealth, or who came in first but by who needed to be treated the most. My dad, clearly in a hurry, wheeled me as quickly as he could to the nearest elevator to take me to the oncology section of the hospital.

When we were entering the elevator, my parents and I ran into someone who used to attend my primary school. This boy was in a wheelchair from birth and physically couldn't walk at all. Meanwhile, I was sitting in a wheelchair because my legs were hurting. At that moment, I saw myself as an imposter. This caused me notable guilt and embarrassment as I felt as though I was mocking the boy or undeserving of the treatment I was receiving. There was light conversation when we first saw each other, however, in the elevator, there was an awkward tension between the boy and his father, me and my parents. I don't think that my parents felt the same sense of embarrassment that I did. Luckily, the elevator trip was only two floors, so I could escape the situation quickly as we left for the oncology department.

In oncology, I was rushed through to a back room that was more comfortable and spacious as a means of mitigating my torment. Rolling through the hallway, I became immersed in a sense of royalty. Everyone and everything were dedicated to my treatment. There were no uncomfortable chairs to sit on in agony for hours as we waited to be seen, and there was no depressing waiting room filled with sick children, their parents overwhelmed by sadness.

The first room I was taken to was a private waiting room with a couch that I could lie down on. I felt relieved as I could sit more comfortably. However, the comfort was short-lived, as the couch could only give me temporary relief, and no sitting position could surmount the burning from within. Not long after that, a nurse approached us. She strapped on a heart rate monitor and took some basic observations. This was how it always worked when I went to the hospital. I would come in, wait hours less than others to be seen, in a room twice as comfortable so that the immunocompromised cancer kid would have limited exposure to other sick people. Then I would have my basic heart rate and blood pressure checked before I was seen by the doctor. We went through the routine questions with the nurse present. "How's the pain? Where is it? Can you describe it? What would you give it on a scale of one to ten?" This felt like a massive redundancy since the doctor would often then ask the exact same questions as soon as they saw me and answering them never seemed to help me. Irrespective of the content of the questions asked, none were helping to ease the fire in my bones at the time.

Five minutes later, the nurse returned with a healthy dose of paracetamol. A minute passed, then two, then five, then 15, but the pain did not subside. After some time had passed, I was able to move into a room with a vacant hospital bed. I could lie down in a more comfortable position, well, as comfortable as possible as I attempted to continue with my schoolwork so as not to fall behind on what my class was currently doing. I made it through the minimum amount I had assigned myself before taking a break. Every time that I took a break from schoolwork during chemo, I was ignited by a palpable sense of hatred for myself, as if I was lazy and undeserving of academic success. I am the kind of person who prides themself on being dedicated to their studies and achieving greatness. Whilst I was still able to achieve academic success off the back of my prior work, which put me so far ahead of my peers, I often felt as though I was not working hard enough. I questioned whether I was taking advantage of the situation I was in, despite knowing that deep down, I was still working harder than most.

In the hospital bed, I was left alone in a room with my parents for an extended period. During such a time, it is important for loved ones to stick together, however, my parents and I could not seem to agree on much. Mum, the paranoid lady she is, was desperate for answers that no one had. Consequently, she turned to the internet to find the answers she was seeking. Unfortunately, this meant engaging in group chats with past cancer survivor parents who all seemed to think that they were doctors themselves and suggested ridiculous, unsupported treatments such as Claratyne (a brand of antihistamine containing the active ingredient loratadine) to treat leg pain. "I think you should try using these medicines, Sebastian. After all, it couldn't hurt." Perplexed by the absurd notion, I criticised my mum. Surely she hadn't just recommended an antihistamine to treat my severe leg pain? I tried to reassure her of the competency of my medical team by explaining the tertiary and field education they had accrued in medicine, yet to no one's surprise, we were unsuccessful in finding common ground. By no means is this meant to be an attack on my mother. She was doing her best in a time when there was a wide variety of unanswered questions, and her actions came from a place of compassion. I figured I could put up with such differences of opinion for a bit longer.

When the oncologists came to my room, they began some basic tests of the mobility of my legs. This involved stretching them, pushing against them and having me push back. The faces of the oncologists revealed what seemed like confusion, but they were hopeful. It was as though the situation in front of them was foreign, yet they knew things would be okay. This was reassuring to me. However, it also told me that I would have to wait a little longer for answers. It even made me doubt myself and whether I was just being overly cautious or weak. Nevertheless, the MRI was finally ordered and as I got up to leave, I was confronted by dozens of little hairs from my legs that had shed onto the hospital bed. At this moment, the realness and magnitude of my situation became apparent. Although confronting, I began to appreciate the challenge of the journey I was on.

The MRI test involved me lying down for a boring hour or so doing nothing in a harsh environment. I didn't mind the discomfort so long as I saw answers. This mentality was consistent throughout many parts of my treatment from before I was even diagnosed to right past the completion of chemo. The results of the MRI would be obtained later via Zoom. One of the many benefits of the pandemic was that the world had become more comfortable communicating online, allowing us to connect in shorter amounts of time whilst limiting unnecessary exposure to sick people. My oncologist, mother and I were all on the Zoom call. The good news was that I would finally receive answers for the pain that I was experiencing.

Sadly, Dr Claira was about to be the bearer of bad news. She diagnosed me with avascular necrosis (AVN), commonly known as osteonecrosis. This condition occurs when the bone (osteo) dies (necrosis) in one's body. For me, this happened throughout many regions of my lower body, including the pelvis, femur, and tibia, but it would later affect many other regions. When receiving the diagnosis, I was surprisingly calm and emotionless. I guess that given everything that was going on at the time, the damage to my bones seemed insignificant, and to be fair, relative to my cancer, they were the least of my worries. When the call ended, I noticed I had the 'whatever' mindset where I just didn't care. It was like, cool, there is now a name for what I'm experiencing, and this would be really intriguing if I was in less pain. Claira also told us that there wasn't any real treatment that was effective against my condition. Thankfully, there was hope it could get better on its own with time. Apart from that, I didn't have to change my lifestyle at all, and I continued to take oxycodone as needed to manage things, but I didn't feel any different. The diagnosis was just words for the pain I was feeling, and I didn't have any strong feelings about what was happening to me at the time. So, with a clear mind, I went straight to my room to relax.

Chapter 12

Chemo Leak

~ *Sebastian* ~

It was the day of my chemo review where I would find out the results of my latest PET-MRI scan. The results of this test would show how my body had responded to the first two rounds of chemotherapy and even dictate my future treatment. The waiting room was calm and lifeless. As per usual, you could feel the pain of the parents around you who were concerned about the welfare of their children. Their concern was warranted, given that at any time one could take a turn for the worse. Meanwhile, many children were blissfully ignorant of the magnitude of their suffering and were quite simply far more concerned with eating McDonald's or playing on their Nintendo Switches. Personally, I was bored. Waiting times to see a doctor are notoriously unfavourable, however, the oncology department takes this to a new level. Given the time-sensitive nature of treating cancer patients, it is paramount that oncologists make use of all of the time available to them to best treat their patients, so they have jam-packed appointment schedules. Whilst I would often attempt to complete some homework during the waits, my attempts would be futile as the environment around me was hardly suitable for working. It was also extremely uncomfortable to hold a computer for an extended period, let alone write in a workbook. Instead, I would succumb to solitude and silence, running down the clock in utter boredom. Finally, after more than an hour, my mum and I would be let in to see the doctor.

 On this particular day, we were receiving critical news about my progress. It meant establishing a firm roadmap to recovery and finding out whether the day would be filled with jubilation or panic. We were immediately sat down in the consultation room. Not the room that we usually sat in, but still a room that we were familiar with. The walls had the same diagrams, the desk had the same computer, and we had the same doctor, yet everything felt completely different. The oncologist faced his computer screen towards us, clearly depicting my prior PET scan results. On one side you could see an outline of myself, brimming with so much metabolic activity that I looked like a Christmas tree on the night of Christmas Eve. Not a visible part of the lymphatic system was without cancer. Alternatively, on the other side of the screen laid a mellow picture, a picture with mere specks of visible metabolic activity that were unlikely to even be cancerous. On the first side, was my initial PET scan results prior to treatment, and on the latter, my current scan.

 In a matter of two months, I had gone from being overwhelmed by uncontrollable proliferating cancer cells, to a boy who could now see the light at the end of the tunnel. There was however a spot around my coccyx bone where there was an increase of metabolic activity. Dr Quinn wasn't sure what it was but informed us that it was unlikely to be of any concern. If it was cancerous, the next four cycles of chemotherapy treatment would surely do the trick. Still, the thought remained, *could it be a cancerous region that wasn't susceptible to the chemo?* I knew that there would still be some cancer cells floating through my body which the next three to four months of chemo should take care of. My family and I would rest a little easier tonight in light of the fantastic news. No longer was the hospital a dull and dark place; to me the hospital now became as lively as a garden bed in the springtime.

Following the review, I would be subjected to a new chemotherapy regimen. Despite the stellar news, I would have to undergo an immensely harsh round of chemo that usually would be used to treat people who didn't respond well to initial rounds of treatment. The reasoning behind this was that this chemo regimen would have less steroids, which would hopefully keep my osteonecrosis at bay as the condition was caused by the steroid prednisolone. The new treatment plan was quite different to what I was used to. In contrast to the five days a week, two-to-four-hour sessions of chemo followed by a few more lone chemo sessions over another week before receiving a fortnight's break, I would now be subjected to four intense days of chemo over the course of a week. For those of you who are curious about what chemotherapy drugs I was receiving, the new plan consisted of cyclophosphamide, etoposide, doxorubicin, prednisolone, vincristine, and dacarbazine. I had prior experience with many of these drugs, however, the new additions would prove to be highly toxic.

It was my first day of the new concoction of medicine, and I would have eight to nine hours of chemo ahead of me. Despite this, before I could start the bulk of the chemo, I needed to ensure that I was well hydrated and this included peeing in a bottle. Every time I used the bathroom, there would be a stack of cardboard bottles there for me, and I would have to pee in one of them. The analysis of the urine sample would indicate how hydrated I was, and whether I was ready to begin receiving the bulk of my chemo. Providing the sample formed a sense of déjà vu that reminded me of the many urine samples I had provided in the lead-up to my diagnosis. The entire process felt primitive and ancient. The shape of the bottle was more like a shoe box than something that would be used to collect urine, and I found it quite counter-intuitive that cardboard would be used to store a liquid substance. Nevertheless, I provided my first sample and went back to completing some schoolwork.

Occasionally, to break up the time that I spent studying, I would be visited by one of the hospital-provided support staff. She was supposed to be tutoring me, but given my high academic standards, she spent far more time playing games with me. One of these games was called *Bananagrams*. The game is a variation of *Scrabble* with no board, where you have a group of letters and try to make words out of them. The support staff member, Betty, would set out the letters in front of me on the hospital bedside table and occasionally Mum would join in. I was undoubtedly the best of the three of us at the game, but Betty and

Sebastian - Chemo Leak

Mum still gave me a run for my money, and on the very rare occasion, beat me. Every time my mum would win, she savoured the moment, and couldn't pass up on the opportunity to rub it in my face. On our Google Home display, photos rotate through of all the times that my mum beat me at *Bananagrams*. I can report that there are not many of these photos!

One day Betty popped in to say hello. It was one of those hospital trips where I spent almost the entire day there. I'd be up with *the early morning chirping of the birds, and in the hospital past the sun's descent beyond the horizon*. Betty figured that I might get bored of doing homework or sitting around and watching TV. She was right. My ability to focus was deteriorating, and it was nice to have the distraction from schoolwork or loneliness.

The nurse would periodically check in to provide us with an update on my hydration. She would say, "You need to keep drinking, Sebastian". The nurse informing me that I wasn't hydrated enough to begin treatment would knock back any confidence that I had left in me. I had tried to stay hydrated through drinking enough, and to be told that you weren't hydrated after all of your efforts was deflating. I was also receiving hydrating fluids that were being pumped into me. Trying to manoeuvre around multiple poles that carried medications and hydrations that ran into my central port every time I went to the bathroom was like a boring course of *Ninja Warrior* with no cash prize for my efforts. Within a couple of hours of being hydrated, I had received all the pre-treatment antiemetic medications and was adequately hydrated, ready for the

The ~~Worst~~ Best Year

long day of chemo ahead of me.

One by one, I received the medicines, flushed through my port. Each medicine was administered in a certain way. Whilst they were also given intravenously, some like dacarbazine had to be covered to mitigate dangerous light exposure, cyclophosphamide required lots of hydration, and then there was doxorubicin, the red devil. This medication had a special machine that was used to administer it. I had become interested in learning about the machines used to administer the chemo and was able to use them to keep track of how long each medication needed to be fully administered. The machine used to administer the doxorubicin would give me a little over 30mLs over an hour. As it was late into the day, I had finished most of my homework and was simply waiting for the chemo to run out. I looked over to see that there were only 3mLs left in the cycle which meant that I was nearing the end of the day as I would only have one to two more drugs left after this treatment. As I turned back to my computer, I felt a tug on the plastic line running into my port (the device used to administer the chemo) and to my surprise, the needle running into my port had become unplugged. The red devil was now going to start leaking onto my skin. BEEP, BEEP, BEEP! The machine had caught on to what was going on.

"Ummm Mum, I think I pulled out the needle. Can you get the nurse?" In a fit of horror, Mum rushed to the door, "Can you help my son? I think he's pulled his port out!"

Now I know that some of you will think that this next bit is exaggerated, but I promise that this felt as surreal as it probably will read. Within seconds, nurses began to rush into my room. In no more than a minute, trained doctors followed with carts containing medicines and equipment. The chemo was stopped, and no more than half a millilitre of the red devil had a chance to leak onto my skin. However, this was enough to cause substantial harm. My dressings on the port were promptly removed and the region was iced. The ice packs, being in the children's oncology ward, were shaped in the form of little animals. Every time I looked up, more nurses and doctors had entered the room. The room was now replete with a dozen medical staff of ranging specialities including oncology, plastic and general surgery in addition to all the nurses nearby. People were scrambling to ensure that protocols had been met when treating such a leak. There was a manual of some sort, a stack of papers stapled together with instructions on how to handle such a chemo leak. The nurses seemed to be reading from the manual, and while it added to the intensity of the moment, it was a little unsettling. One nurse handed me a new ice pack with a picture of a panda on it. It must have been the third or fourth ice pack I was now on. I needed to keep changing them out in the hope of keeping the affected area optimally iced and protected until I was properly treated.

Within 15 minutes of the initial leak, I found myself on the other side of the oncology ward receiving some nitrous oxide to help alleviate the pain that I was about to experience as a result of the emergency procedure that was underway. Interestingly, the procedure occurred in one of the rooms that is usually used to access people's ports. I ended up becoming high on laughing gas. The affected region around the site of my port was further numbed before a fine and long needle was injected into the area, piercing the skin with ease. Fluid was pushed through the needle to flush the region of any doxorubicin to minimise any long-term damage. That needle was followed by two dozen more all in the same region in a slightly different position that attempted to achieve the same purpose. Even with the pain relief medication that I had received, the pain was still present. Not as bad as the osteonecrosis that I had previously experienced, but definitely not as simple as a routine blood test. I was glad to be awake for the procedure as even though the medication I had received was supposed to interfere with my memory, I have a feeling that I might be remembering this better than my high school graduation a decade from now.

Occasionally, one of the needles would catch me by surprise or hit a region that was less heavily medicated, and you could visibly see my facial reaction to the pain. However, as I was high on gas, I made humour out of the situation. I likely distracted the medical team more than I should have, given that they were trying to carry out a medical procedure. In my less than mentally sound state, I would make a wide-mouthed facial expression as the needle would hit my skin, not because I couldn't bear the pain, but because I'd thought it would be funny to see the procedure from my mum's perspective. The gas had taken over my sensibleness and all I wanted to do was capture that very moment and keep the memory alive. Hence, the very high version of me thought it would be a good idea to ask my mum to take a photo of the surgery whilst it was taking place. "Take a photo, Mum. Take a photo, Mum." I

Sebastian - Chemo Leak

also asked that she capture the procedure on video footage, but I was unsuccessful with that request (I still do think a video would have been nice though).

I noticed one of the nurses completing some administrative work. There was a computer with my file on it which included statistics of my medical history and current observations of my medical state. There were plenty of boxes to enter information into, although I was more drawn to the diagram of a person who was presumably depicting me. The diagram was plain, a simple outline of a person. That struck me as unusual and so I was wondering, if this was supposed to be a picture of a man, then where the heck was my, well, you know, thing between the legs? The gas was still very clearly taking its effect on me, and in my heightened state, I enquired on the matter. Surprised, the nurse gave a slight chuckle, and my mum followed suit. Having endured this experience was not going to make me stronger in spirit but was going to provide me with an interesting story to tell. In the days, weeks, and months to follow, I would tell people about the time I pulled my needle out and Mum would tell the story about the time her son had 'burnt' himself while receiving chemo. I also didn't fail to take my own photos of the aftermath, with dozens of bruises left behind from the procedure.

Spending the night in observation at the hospital was an inevitable outcome, which meant I would be able to see a new part of the hospital. Periodically, throughout the night, nurses would come in to check on me, and plastic surgeons would inspect the region where the surgery was conducted. It was later in the night when my oncologist came

The ~~Worst~~ Best Year

to visit. I lifted up my shirt so that he could inspect my port and he started searching for discolouration. The unfazed look on his face and slight smile signified to me that all looked good. The doxorubicin had failed to cause any long-term damage. "I have some news. We are all good to continue chemo tomorrow," he informed. On a day filled with a rollercoaster of emotions like a *bouncy ball* rolling down a street, I was content to know that the future was steady, and I was back on track. With the fear and pain of the day behind me, it was time to celebrate the fact that I was moving forward and making progress in a huge battle against cancer.

It would not come to be your typical party. I felt pretty normal, which was contrary to the concern from my family. Mum made many phone calls to inform people of the great news. Alongside the calls, she filled her journal with the emotions that she had experienced while enduring the many events of that day. When I was first diagnosed, my mum was emotionally distraught, and recording her thoughts in a journal seemed to be helpful for her. I think she wanted to remember her emotions, and experiences. She may have felt as though she had missed out on the opportunity to do this when she had cancer. The journalling would continue throughout my journey with cancer, and even after chemotherapy had been completed. I would often wonder what it was she was writing about. Whenever she was frustrated with me, or with life, the pen would come out and it was time for her to let out her frustrations on whoever and whatever she wanted to, with the power of her pen. The only issue I had with this was that my family and I didn't always know what Mum was upset about when she was writing. When she screamed and argued (the best kind of communication), at least we knew what was wrong as it revealed her emotions to us. When she would write in her journal, no one would know what she was thinking, who she was upset with, why she was upset, and what could be done to rectify the situation.

I spent a large portion of my cancer treatment trying to be left alone, but when I expressed this to my family, I was portrayed as a villain. Putting up with others wanting to see and talk to me or check in on me to see how I was going proved to be rather exhausting. However, I knew it was going to be a repetitive norm as long as I was sick, so I had to put up with it. For another few months, I had to endure the well-meaning prodding and poking from 99% of the people I was close with. There were only a handful of people who bucked the trend. These few saw me as a whole person and were prepared to make adjustments to accommodate me without overtly involving themselves with my life at a time when I was overwhelmed by a swarm of concerns.

One of them, whom many called my twin, never uttered the C-word to me. He was the kind of person that you wanted around when you craved normality. The last thing you wanted to hear was yet another, "Are you okay Sebastian?" when you already had a thousand people asking you that. My old year-level coordinator also never liked talking about my treatment, although he did everything that he could to help me. If he did ask, it was in a 'are you all good?' way rather than, 'spill the goss'. The genuine nature of it made me feel like he cared about me.

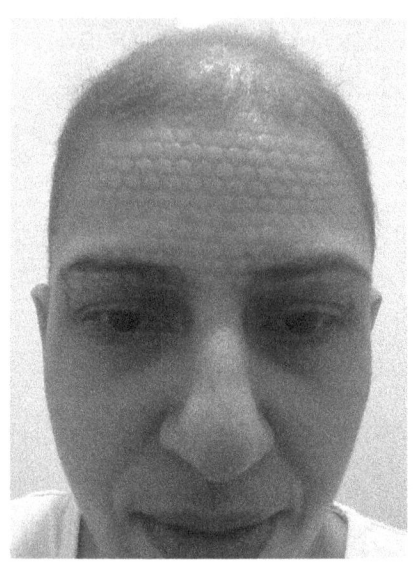

Natalie - Radiation mask imprint, The imprint stayed visible for an hour after each treatment.

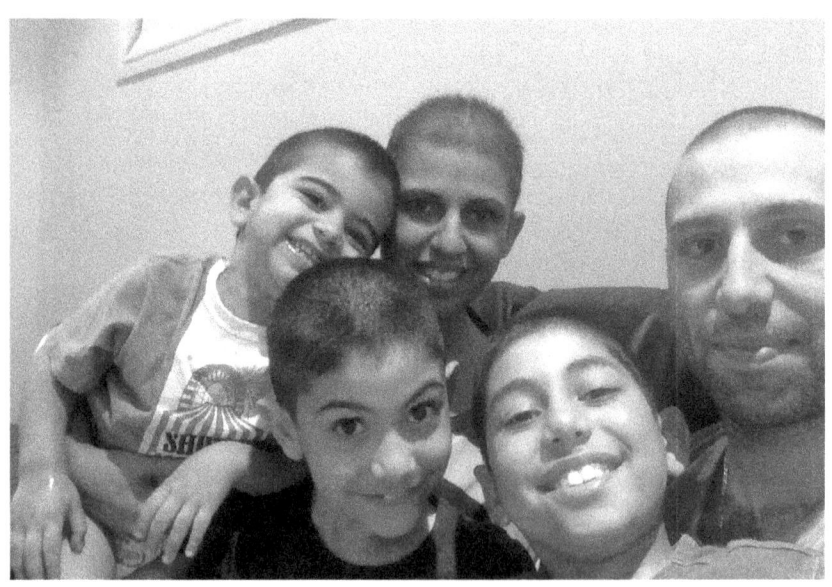

Supporting Natalie through treatment - the first time Elijah, Sebastian, Jerome and George wore the 'team uniform'.

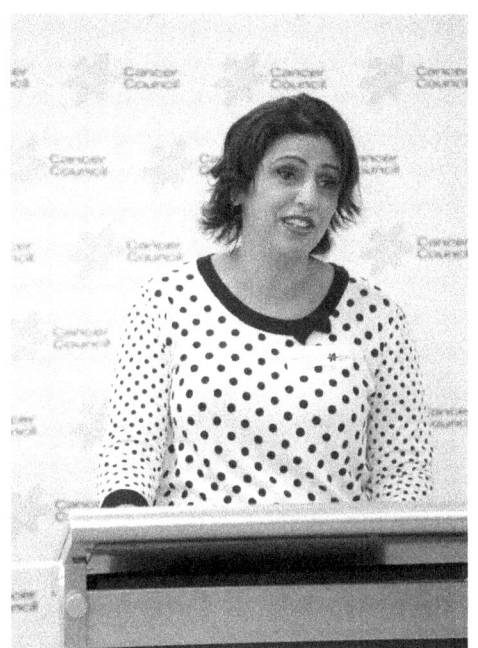

Natalie's first public speech as Ambassador for the Cancer Council.

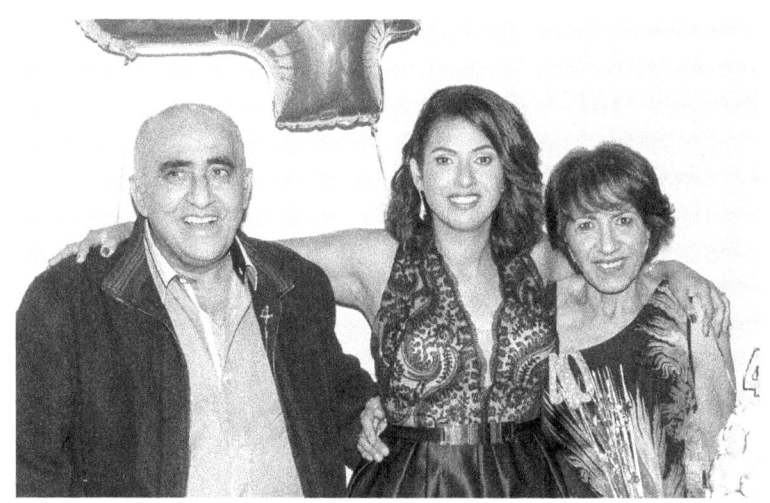

Natalie with her mother and late father at her 40th birthday party.

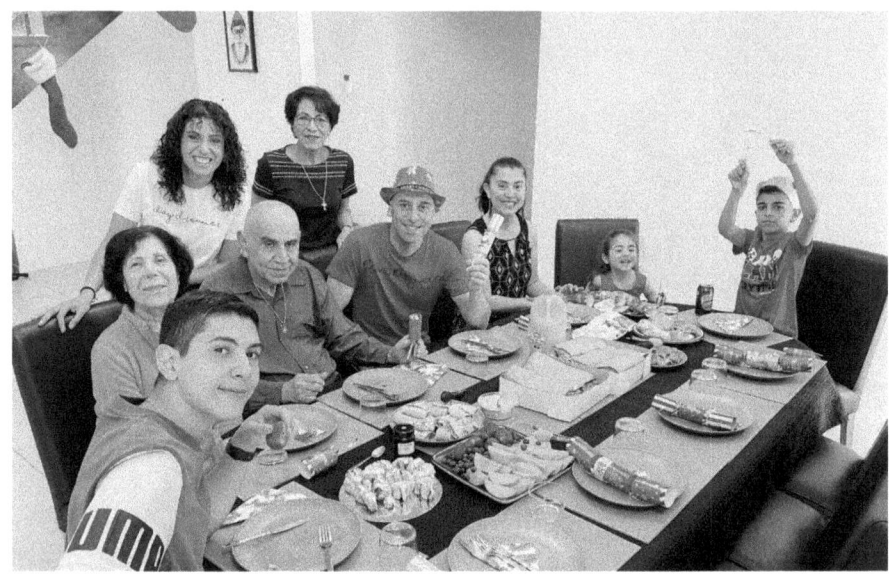

Happy times - Christmas 2021, just before Sebastian's diagnosis with the grandparents, Aunty Gladys and cousin Sarah.

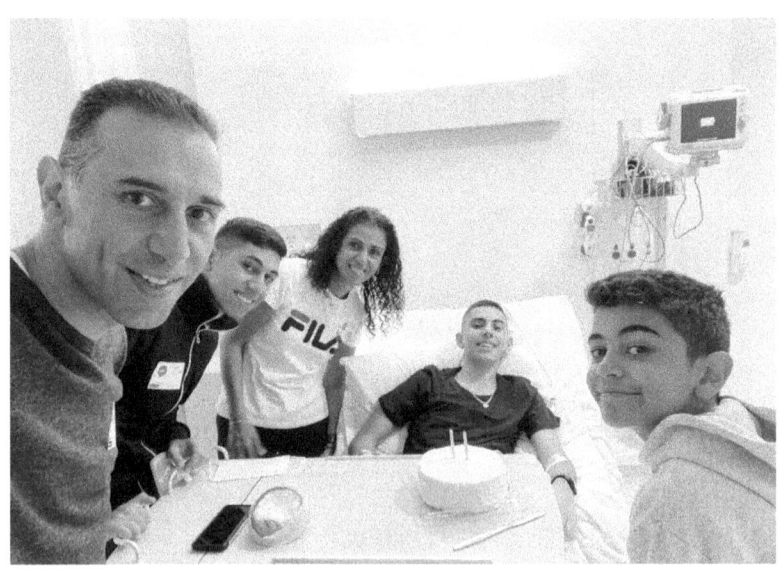

Good Friday 2022. First chemotherapy on Elijah's 11th birthday.

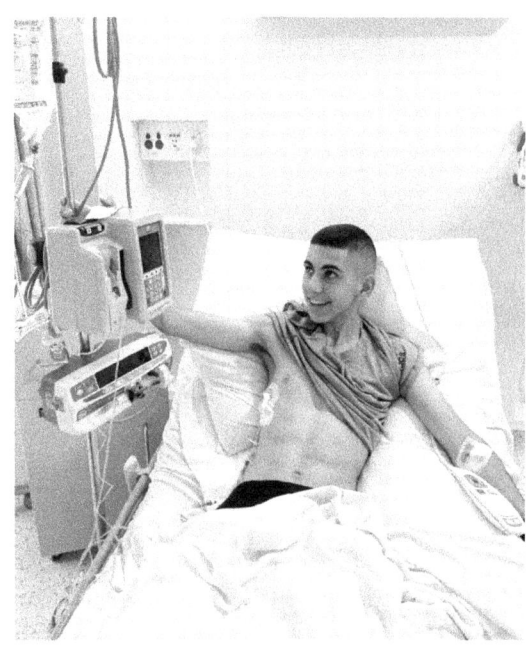

Day one of chemotherapy, a day full of mixed emotions.

Natalie winning Bananagrams, a rare moment captured.

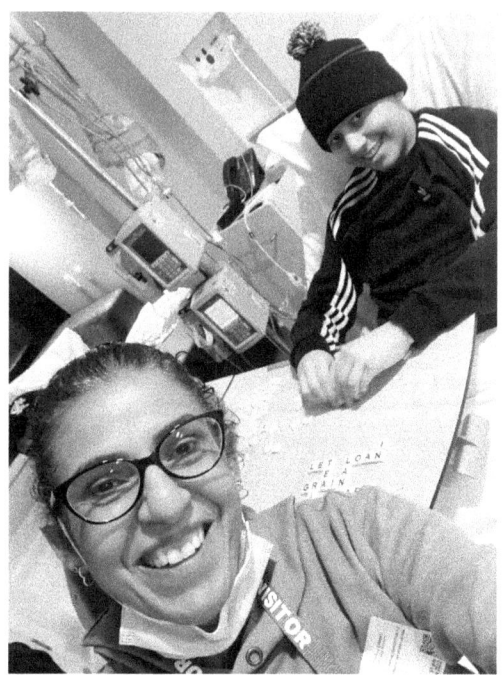

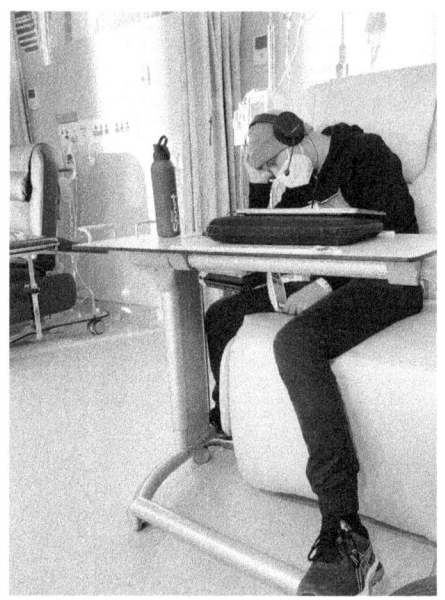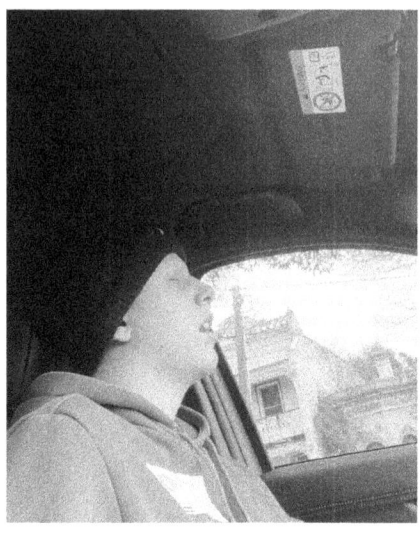

Motivation to study was a great distraction during chemotherapy, and sometimes a nap helped get through. But some days were harder than others, especially on back-to-back chemo days.

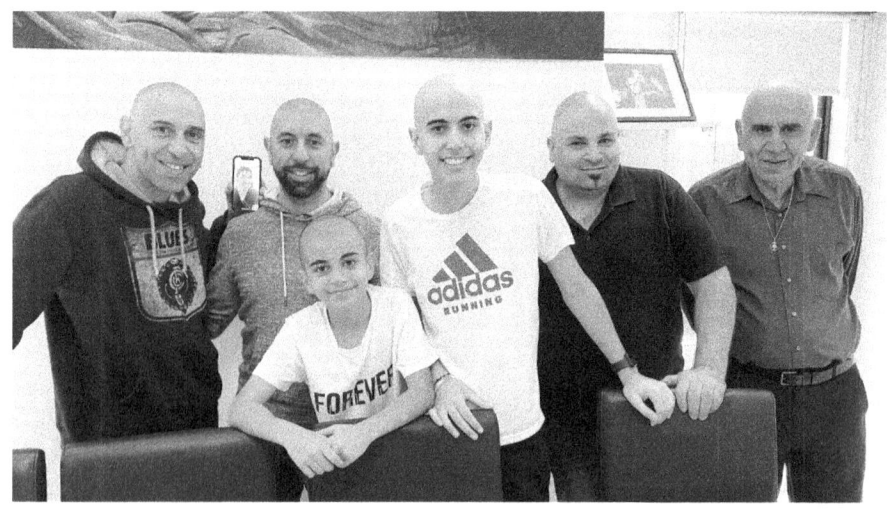

Khoury boys in team uniform, including Jerome on FaceTime isolating with COVID at his grandmother's house.

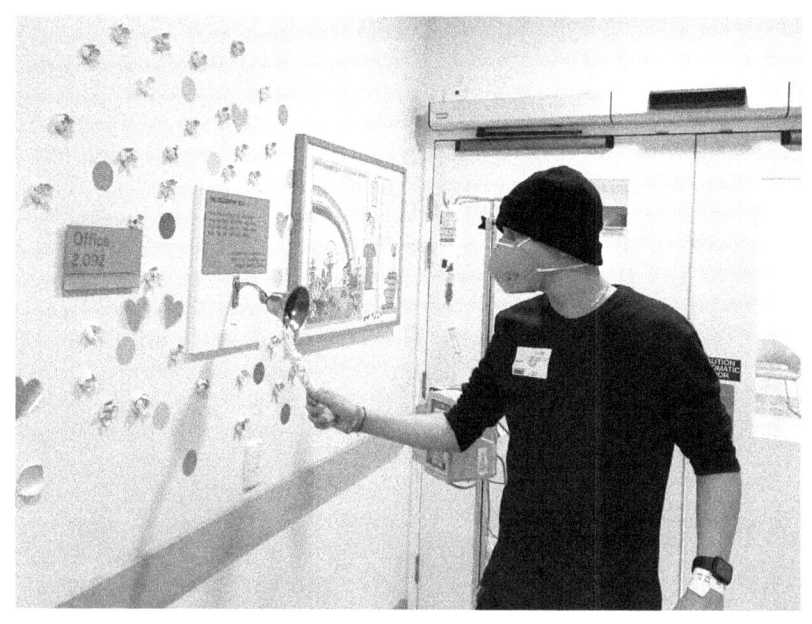

Best sound in the world, ringing the bell symbolising the end of chemotherapy.

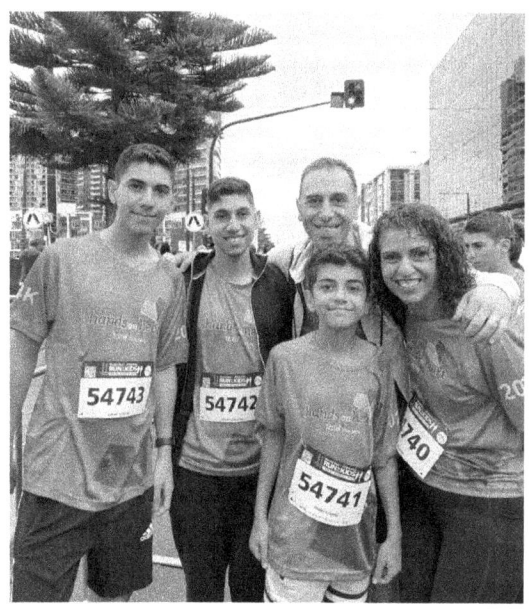

Run for The Kids 2023.

Chapter 13

Cancer And Personal Life

~ Sebastian ~

Attending school with cancer was interesting, to say the least, although I did spend the majority of the time learning from home. It was as if the pandemic lockdown had extended, but this time, only for me. The school was extremely supportive, putting processes in place to support me physically and emotionally. I completed online learning for the larger portion of another year just as I had done the past two years in the thick of the pandemic. One difference between my learning journey during cancer as opposed to that of the pandemic, was the reduced level of accountability. I found it more challenging to exceed my usual excellence than I had in the past as no one had any expectations of me. In a world where everyone expects you to be a genius, you tend to find motivation to work hard so that you meet those expectations. However, in a world where people only expect you to sit in bed and 'recover', that is often all you are motivated to do. When one is nothing more than a *bald head,* they have a restricted view of what they can achieve.

    I would often sleep in and watch TV until 9:30 in the morning, whilst my peers at school would already be halfway through their first period. I was able to ensure that I got all my work done by the end of the school day, but I focussed mostly on maths and business management since they were VCE (Year 11) subjects. The only exception to this was when I had an assessment task due, and I worked hard for a few days to ensure I kept my grades up. Overall, my level of motivation had dwindled substantially compared to what it was a mere few months prior.

    In every cycle of chemo, which usually lasted around three to four weeks, I would try and return to school on a few occasions. If I couldn't stay for the entire school day, I'd attend half days at least. I sometimes would arrive at recess and stay for the rest of the day or come in for my more important subjects like maths methods and business in the morning, and then leave at lunchtime. There was no set schedule to this and it was determined by how I was feeling at the time.

    I remember one treacherous night when I was suffering from insomnia, likely connected to the fact that I was on a very high dose of the steroid prednisolone. I had awoken at 2:00 am after only falling asleep a few hours prior. After trying to get to sleep for three hours the night before and failing, I decided to open YouTube, found a playlist of old videos in a series and watched that series until 9:00 am. There was also another night that I recall when I woke up at 2:00 am and didn't even attempt to return to sleep. I seized the chance to watch YouTubers who I hadn't watched in years, enjoying their old videos that had me initially

The ~~Worst~~ Best Year

hooked. It was actually really fun doing crazy things like binge-watching a series for seven hours straight to relive my nostalgic memories. There aren't many points in your life where you have the luxury to do that when you want to and so I embraced the opportunities as they came.

Being on the school's campus did not come without its perks. First of all, I was given the honour of wearing a beanie at school despite the school having a strict policy at the time that forbade it. I know, big whoop for me. I would try to head off to school on days I felt well and had minimal other commitments. After living at home with no one expecting much of me for such a long time, I experienced a state of motivational inertia where I was far less motivated to work hard and come to school than I normally would be. However, I still managed to attend where I could since my brain thrived on the benefits of productivity, something I had missed out on for extended periods during my cancer journey. Every time I spent a few hours watching TV, I would think about how much more productive I could have been, and all that I could have learned in that time. This would eat away at me and make me hate myself as I chose to complete the bare minimum.

Entering the school gates was a daunting experience. Upon walking through the front gate, I felt like an outsider. I looked different to everyone else with my beanie and hairless appearance standing out among the other students. People would be eager to see and talk to me. They had many questions regarding my health and what it was like for me to go through cancer. Overwhelmingly, people were immensely supportive, complimenting me on my bravery and success despite the setbacks I had faced. While no one intentionally treated me in a negative manner when interacting with me, it was clear that some were more unaware of my condition, despite it being spoken about within and outside of my high school quite frequently. Those who were a little less aware found themselves quite embarrassed from time to time. Even though word of my condition had managed to spread across Melbourne like wildfire, some people in my homeroom at school would occasionally question me on why I was wearing a beanie or why I was spending so much time away from school.

When I was faced with these sorts of questions, it was easiest to provide an answer that wasn't necessarily specific to cancer such as wearing a beanie "to keep my head warm" or being away from school because "I was sick". This way I could avoid getting caught up in an uncomfortable conversation where they would feel guilty for asking such questions in the first place. Another bonus was that this was a very authentic 'Sebastian' kind of smart-ass comment to remind everyone that just because I was sick, didn't mean that I was not still me.

It wasn't just the odd student that failed to get the memo. Some teachers, despite being emailed about a student in my year having cancer and being allowed to wear a beanie, seemed to keep asking me to take it off as it wasn't part of the school uniform. They were oblivious to the fact that I was the student in the school who had cancer. In such a case, humour was my friend. Faced with the options of explaining that I was the kid with cancer, or just obeying their request, I often chose the latter, intrigued by how they would react when they realised that they had just asked a sick, bald, child to take off their beanie. Once a teacher had made such a mistake the first time, they tended to think twice before asking again. Moreover, each time that a teacher did accidentally tell me to take the beanie off, they seemed to feel quite guilty and then proceeded to have a five-minute conversation with me with the customary, "How's the treatment going?", almost to prove that they weren't heartless people.

Whilst toying with them was an extremely enjoyable way to spend my time between classes at school, nothing topped that time before homeroom when I wasn't the one to remove the beanie. Following a treacherous cycle of chemotherapy, I once again found myself on the school campus, catching up with friends on what we had missed out on in the time we were apart. This was a particularly enjoyable experience for me since it allowed me to be 'normal' again. I could interact with people in a way where I wasn't the kid with cancer, but just a friend. On this particular occasion, I was able to catch up with my friends outside our homeroom. My friend Connor was relishing the chance to tell me all the stories and mishaps that occurred in my absence. Every Monday morning when I saw him, I looked forward to hearing what craziness he had invited into his life over the weekend, while my head was buried in books and living a relaxed life. This particular day, Connor had my friend Zac and me invested in his story when I felt a little pinch on the top of my head, and realised my beanie had come completely off in front of more than a dozen students.

Now, I didn't care that my beanie had been removed, and I would often take it off in class when I was hot or moving around outside. I also wore the beanie out of comfort and as to not disturb the little children who weren't accustomed to my bald look, not just to keep my head warm. Assuming the beanie didn't just fall off on its own and pairing that with the fact I felt the pinch, it was clear that someone else took it off. I figured it was probably a friend of mine and so I turned around ready to shake the kid's hand and say "Hey!" To my surprise, I was greeted by a teacher who thought it would be a funny idea to take off my beanie thinking I was just a kid out of uniform. While I found the situation amusing, this teacher, who I had never seen before, became as red as a tomato as he realised what he had just done. He was showing all tones of utter embarrassment, with him frozen still, not knowing what to say or do. The thing that made the situation worse was that he was still holding my beanie in his hand and was too awkward to know what to do with it. After a couple of seconds of contemplation, he quickly handed the beanie back, gave me a quick "sorry mate" and ran out the nearest exit before I even had time to react.

Not everyone was able to recognise me when I was sick, and while it hurt to slowly transform into a new person and have no control over it, I never once lost the laugh in me. Whilst much of my family had come to see me since my diagnosis for a customary visit, by the third month of treatment, I was still getting visits from some people who hadn't seen me since my diagnosis. When I first started treatment, thin patches of hair would come out as I played with my hair while watching TV. Eventually, the hairs on my legs came out in my bed. By this point,

The ~~Worst~~ Best Year

I was looking like one of the least hairy Lebanese boys you would ever see; Connor artfully described this as my "woman legs" whenever he saw me at school. I only had a few whiskers on my eyebrows and that was it. I wore a beanie and glasses around the house, and my face had rounded, making me hardly recognisable to someone who hadn't seen me in a while.

While my phone still allowed me to unlock it with Face ID, not everyone could tell the difference. Our family Google Photos account, which grouped photos by the people in it, had automatically created a separate person. When you would click on these photos, they were all of me from when I had started treatment. I had obviously changed enough for it to think that I was a new person. On this particular day, one of my old co-workers, Chloe, had decided to come and visit me. It felt like a lifetime ago that I was in the pizza shop running around and living my normal life, yet it had only been a couple of months. Chloe would often work the same weekend shifts as me and take me home whenever we finished at the same time. Whenever we were both on, I just knew it was going to be a fun shift, and we worked really well together.

When she arrived, she greeted my mum at the door, while I stayed cozied up on our couch. It was her first time seeing a lot of my family so she began to introduce herself to them one by one, until she got to me. Something seemed a little different when she looked at me. Chloe would usually have an infectious smile whenever she saw me, but this felt a little odd, like she was unsure about something. Was it because

Sebastian - Cancer And Personal Life

I was wearing a beanie and was going through so much? Did she just feel bad for me and not know how to express it? Did she not want to get too close to me and make me sick? Then she said, "Hi, I'm Chloe". To which I sarcastically responded, "Hi, I'm Sebastian". Her face dropped as it clicked in her head what had just happened. Apparently, after ten weeks of chemo, I had become unrecognisable, even to her.

***

The times at school during chemo were some of the best moments of the journey. Whilst nothing beats the special and unique memories formed on my trips to the hospital in a once-in-a-lifetime experience, returning to school brought about emotions that were in a league of their own. Towards the end of my cancer journey, after I had spent many months largely learning remotely, I was blessed with the opportunity to be welcomed back into the school by my peers and teachers. Every time people saw me, they wanted to know how I was going, and if I was making improvements; they wanted to be a part of my life. Walking into a class made me feel powerful. After a little while of not being in that class, I would be greeted with cheers, and people just wanting to hear how I had been. I was that special person, and I didn't even do anything.

In typical Sebastian style, I casually walked into class one day after having just spent the last week and a half learning from home. As soon as the teacher arrived, I sat down at the front near my mates and pulled out my MacBook. I was genuinely excited to be there and I was able to experience normalcy which I enjoyed. We were completing

The ~~Worst~~ Best Year

physics as part of the science course. We were learning about distance, displacement, velocity, and many other like terms before using them in calculations. The teacher drew little maps on the board with windy turns. It was our job to calculate the distance, which was the amount of space travelled and displacement, which was the shortest distance between any two positions. I found the work simple, which allowed me to just enjoy being back in the classroom.

Chapter 14

The COVID Holiday

~ *Sebastian* ~

I always hated waking up feeling sick. When you get up in the morning feeling slightly thirsty, only to realise that it's a sore throat, which is only going to inevitably get worse. I was seven weeks into treatment and I hadn't been too sick, but I knew that I was not getting off this easily and I'd soon find my way into the RCH Emergency Department. When Mum entered my room to check in on me, I asked for a Rapid Antigen Test (RAT) so I could test for COVID. We were lucky enough to have a stockpile of tests in storage that were enough to last another six-month lockdown should we need to. These were from all the free ones that the government and our school were giving out like boxes of chocolate at Easter. We had moved past the point of reading the instructions on the labels of the RATs even though each brand had slightly different ones. Instead, we would just swab each nostril somewhere between five and ten times before placing it in the

The ~~Worst~~ Best Year

solution, mixing it around, waiting a minute and then squeezing the solution onto the testing strip. It perplexed me how we managed before the home RATs, when we were subjected to days of anticipation and anxiety waiting to find out our test results as if it was a teacher marking a school exam. Thank goodness we had moved past that.

Since I had to give the test 10-15 minutes before checking it, I thought I would watch some TV. My parents had installed a TV in my room when I started treatment since they figured I would be spending a lot of time in my room and it came in handy, especially during times like these. Just shy of my bed width, nothing too fancy, but enough to get me through. Nowadays this is more of a curse, making it too easy to waste time watching TV on the weekends. Sometimes, I might even hide the batteries for the remote somewhere in my room to discourage me from watching TV, but that never lasts. My brother had caught COVID only a week prior and he was instantly shipped off to my grandmother's house to isolate for a week as per *Khoury protocol*. So, it was unlikely that I caught COVID from him, although it was a possibility as I became sick soon after his return.

About time to check on the rapid test, I thought. My hand tremored as I picked the test up and took a glance. Although only a very faint line was present, it still indicated a positive test result and it was time to call the hospital. There was a dedicated oncology 'fast track' number which allowed you to speak to a specialised team during treatment. My mum rang this number more than she rang my grandmother. They instructed us to come straight into the hospital to complete a PCR test which would confirm the result, as RATs were not as accurate as the PCR tests. To do this, we needed to be careful. In our household, we were always careful. COVID, cancer, or a seasonal flu, Mum's paranoia could not be tamed. When one of us caught COVID, we would often isolate ourselves at my grandmother's house. This was mainly to protect me from getting sick during treatment. If we were isolating at home, the person isolating would be in our spare bedroom downstairs. We would have our own private bathroom and a lining under the door to prevent any transmission of illness. Someone would drop off food to them via the bathroom entrance with an N95 mask and that was the closest they came to contact. When the isolating person picked up their food, they would also wear an N95 to prevent any COVID viruses from leaving the isolation room. It worked very well and we rarely if ever transmitted COVID when the *Khoury Protocols* were in place.

    The PCR test at the hospital was conducted in their parking section. On the road stood a construction sign that read 'COVID-19 testing'. Turning into the parking area led us down a path filled with twists and turns like a mini obstacle course. The turns probably weren't a great idea when considering that the people who were driving through were often sick and nauseous to begin with. There weren't too many cars lined up in the parking lot, so someone came to our car door promptly to enquire about our details. The person at the other end of the oncology fast track phoneline had told us to tell them that we were from the oncology ward of the hospital. This was like a superpower since the hospital prioritises the treatment of cancer patients given the severity of the sickness and the need to minimise patients contracting any further illnesses. When we told them that I was from the oncology ward, they promised to rush my test.

Someone dressed in full personal protective equipment (PPE) shortly approached my car door to administer the test. It's hard to forget the feeling of having a swab inserted so far up your nostrils that it felt like the swab touched the back of your head. Anyone who lived through the pandemic would remember how annoying it was to have their nose swabbed. Just for good measure, they gave us a handful of extra tests for free as they do when you get a PCR test; no wonder our stockpiles were overcapacity. What amazed me was that a mere few months earlier, you would be paying $10.00 per test; now, they were being thrown away by the dozens. The rush on the test was quite fast. Rather than waiting in excess of a day like others at the time, the hospital was able to confirm my diagnosis in a couple of hours.

I was now left with a choice to either go downstairs to the Khoury isolation room or isolate in my room upstairs. I didn't stay at my grandmother's house, since my grandmother wasn't in the best position to help me should a cancer-related issue arise when I was at her house. My room was positioned well enough with proximity to the bathroom to also serve as an isolation room. There was a minimal risk of getting Jerome in the room opposite to me sick as he had just recently recovered from COVID. Plus, I had my TV in my room which meant that it would be far more comfortable to isolate there. I had an ongoing date with Netflix for the entire week. I was buried under layers

Sebastian - The COVID Holiday

of warmth, curled up in my bed with no one to disturb me.

Except my mum who kept ringing to check in on me. Every half an hour, I had to check my temperature to see if I had hit 38°C. The hospital mandated that any kid receiving chemo with a temperature of 38°C or higher had to come into the emergency ward for treatment to prevent serious illness. I had so far refrained from going to the hospital even if I knew I was sick before now since I didn't want to put extra strain on the hospital system if the illness was only mild. Unfortunately, even what would normally constitute a very mild disease could easily progress to a more severe disease when my immunity was suppressed during chemotherapy treatment. I checked my temperature, and I was at 36.8°C. Back to watching some Netflix. While watching *Friends* reruns got me through the pain in my legs, I was going to need a new show for this week. It took a little while to find one, but I got there eventually. I always loved the feeling of starting a new TV series that had half a dozen seasons. There was almost a peace of mind that your entertainment needs were going to be covered for the next little while. My next check-in with the thermometer saw the temperature break 37°C and it wouldn't be long before we hit 38°C. My temperature would usually sit in the mid to high 35°C range with the home thermometer, so even the mid 36°Cs would mean I wasn't far off a trip to the hospital. I started preparing for a trip to the Emergency Department and I hit 37.8°C within only ten minutes before calling Mum to tell her it was time.

The car was loaded with luggage for the hospital trip and my family made way for me to not get too close as I walked downstairs and entered the car. We gave the RCH a call on the fast-track number so they could prepare for our arrival. The ride to the hospital would not be short of precautions either. I was layered with an N95 mask and face shield, whilst my mum had the same. I was on the opposite side of the car in the back seat, furthest from Mum to maximise our distance. As my temperature was rapidly rising, my arms and jaw frantically started to shiver. The excruciating drive to the hospital would take about 20 minutes, which was not ideal when you're shivering to your core. On top of this, Mum kept all the windows open to let a breeze in, which assisted in further preventing the spread of COVID. However, this also exacerbated my shivering, making the journey exponentially more challenging. Jumper, pants, cuddled up in a ball, nothing would calm the shivering. I was going to be stuck like this for a while until my body thought I was hot enough. Mum went in, told the receptionist my details, and that I was COVID-positive while I waited at a safe distance. A double-whammy. Not only did I have cancer, but I had COVID so surely my treatment was going to be extra fast now.

Given the circumstances, I was immediately rushed to the nearest room to separate myself from all the other sick kids so as not to make them sicker or even get myself more sick. I had my beanie on at the time which may have artificially elevated my temperature to the ear temperature checker the hospital used, although when they checked, the 39.4°C they recorded was undoubtedly a cause for concern. The nurse asked the basic questions about symptoms, so I gave her a short summary of this chapter so far. It wasn't too long before we ended up

Sebastian - The COVID Holiday

in a negative pressure room (an isolation room where the air pressure inside the room is lower than the air pressure outside the room) whilst waiting for a spot to open up on the wards. The negative pressure helped to keep air from flowing out of the room when nurses and doctors entered to check in on me or give me medicine, to minimise the ward's exposure to the pathogens I was carrying. The hospital was constantly dealing with spacing and too many patients, but they always seemed to find a way for the sickest patients to be treated.

It had been a long day, and my mum was hungry. The nurses had dropped off some sandwiches and Mum didn't mind them but they were a struggle for me to eat. She asked my dad to drop off some food at the hospital. There was a kebab shop and a KFC that were close by, and he was on his way. Mum asked what I wanted and we decided KFC chips and chicken was enough to satiate our hunger. We spent the time sitting around and talking to family. Mum was taking photos of me in the hospital bed, to show everyone that I was doing well. My aunty was constantly video calling us during my treatment, with my little cousin Sarah on the call with her. She often called Mum and me via video to check in. Mum would turn the phone around to face me, not knowing that you could just press a button on your screen to rotate the screen. Sarah would always be running around the house trying to show us what she had made, or toys that she liked. This meant we spent most of the time looking at shaky footage while my aunty chased her around the house until she was so fatigued that she lost her breath, which never seemed to get old no matter how many times it happened.

The ~~Worst~~ Best Year

It sparked my curiosity about how people saw me when I had cancer. I didn't particularly worry about them seeing me weak, but I did find it fascinating how they perceived me during times like this. Was I a suffering kid or was I 'Seb the witty teenager'; maybe I was both. Dad soon called to inform us that he had dropped off the food at the front to be passed onto us, and it wasn't long before a nurse in full PPE uniform brought it in. Mum and I took turns eating: one would be masked while the other ate, and then we switched. Obviously, I would be expelling COVID particles that would linger in the air even after I put my mask back on, but it would be safer this way (or at least it gave us the perception that we were safe). I must not have been too hungry because I barely made it through the chips, before becoming uninterested in eating anymore. I sat and relaxed, scrolling on my phone while we waited and waited for a room to become available.

Eventually, Mum wanted to get the nurse, but we couldn't really just walk out into the Emergency Department when she had just spent the day with COVID-positive me and the hallways were festering with sick children. I don't recall why she wanted the nurse; it was for something trivial anyway. The nurse call button was part of the TV remote which was typically attached to the hospital bed via a white, windy cord. The only problem was that we couldn't find this cord for some reason, so she took things into her own hands. She figured that the help button on the wall would contact the nurse, so pressed it. The issue was that she had unknowingly managed to press the emergency button which signified to the medical team in the triage section of the medical department that I was in profound medical distress. Straight away, we could hear a kerfuffle outside my room.

Within 15 seconds a fleet of medical staff were suited up and stormed into our isolation room in full PPE, busting through the door fully prepared for anything. They immediately asked my mum what happened, and she told them that she needed their help, not realising that she had just sounded the emergency alarm. They almost seemed disappointed as if it was so bad that I wasn't going into cardiac shock or worse. In their defence, it would be quite annoying to go through all that effort for nothing. When they told us that she had pressed the emergency button she was quite apologetic. I recall laughing our heads off throughout the remainder of the night and occasionally in the months to come. We added this story to the repertoire of funny cancer mishaps.

A few hours passed as we waited, until we were eventually moved up into the cancer ward by a nurse's escort. We were put into the negative pressure room of the ward, again to help prevent COVID particles from leaving my room and infecting cancer patients. Mum was determined to stay with me throughout my stay, and so it took all of my might to convince her to return home. The doctors told her that she could drop anything off to me, but if she left, she couldn't come back. They also said that if she caught COVID when staying with me, she would have to leave if she was too sick to stay. This almost convinced her to stay, had I not begged her otherwise. I partly wanted her to leave so she did not become sick but mainly wanted some peace and quiet.

Irrespective of my intentions, she eventually agreed to leave. Before

The ~~Worst~~ Best Year

she did, she begged me to take my mask off despite having COVID and all the precautions she had made me take all day to avoid her getting sick. Now I get that she didn't want the mask to leave impressions on my face, but I found it perplexing that she was so cautious one minute, wearing N95 face masks and face shields, sitting on the opposite side of the car with the windows rolled down on the freeway, to only a couple of hours later wanting me to take my mask off metres away from her. Nevertheless, by midnight she was gone and so too was her stressing.

That night, I struggled to sleep while enduring the shiver-sweat cycles and headaches from high temperatures along with a sore throat. I also woke up many times throughout the night to nurses coming in and giving me medication at random hours in short bursts rather than all at once. The benefit of being in the hospital though was that the nurses only came in when they needed to, which was less often than what I would have dealt with at home.

The next morning, I flicked on the TV to pass the time and switched things up every so often with some YouTube on the computer. I had nothing to do all day except FaceTime with Mum when the oncologist came in for their rounds, as she made me promise to do so before she left. The only real hassle was trying to move around and take care of my IV machine. Since I had to unplug and replug the charging cables each time I stood up, it made moving around annoying. I would also have to carefully navigate the machine around corners in the room and to the bathroom without getting it caught in anything which was a challenge, time-consuming, and tedious at times. The day went by quickly with few distractions. The oncologist came in at midday. As for the COVID, I had a sore throat, headache, and some temperature fluctuations, but it didn't feel too severe. There were only a few times when the temperature spiked past 39°C and I wasn't feeling too well, however, I spent a large portion of my day enjoying the silence.

When Dr Cooper, the oncology fellow on duty, came in, I told him about how my mum was forcing me to FaceTime her, and he didn't seem too surprised. Maybe a lot of parents were as crazy as my mum, and he was used to it by then. He told me that he wasn't too concerned about my COVID. To prevent the disease from becoming too severe, though, I would be given Paxlovid. Paxlovid consisted of ritonavir and nirmatrelvir. The nirmatrelvir would act as the inhibitor which prevented the survival and replication of coronaviruses whilst ritonavir would enhance this effect. I had to begin the prescription quickly as antiviral medication such as this works most effectively to prevent severe disease when prescribed proactively and quickly. Given the enhancing effect of ritonavir, I would have to postpone chemo for a week until the Paxlovid had cleared my system so as not to impact the effects of the chemo treatment.

I spent the rest of the day on my computer while my phone charged on the other side of the room, until I heard my mum talking. I am not kidding when I tell you that she started talking to me out of nowhere and I wasn't going crazy. In fact, it was Mum who had gone crazy. Somehow, she had managed to call the nurse in charge of the ward, get the room that I was in and the phone number to it. Rather than the

The ~~Worst~~ Best Year

phone ringing through, it had a feature enabled which meant that it would automatically answer calls. Therefore, Mum could call whenever she wanted and startle me. If she annoyed me enough, I could have just unplugged the phone, which I came quite close to doing. Turns out, she just wanted to check in on me, as well as have a go at me for not answering her phone call which never came through on my phone. So, I returned to relaxing and passing the time until my next meal.

Hospital meals were not appealing. You would order through a website, and there was a range of choices, but the meals were all mass-produced, often soggy, and tasted revolting which meant that I often ate quite minimally in the hospital. Knowing I felt this way, Mum offered to bring me some leftover Lebanese food from a restaurant that they were eating out at, which made for a wonderful dinner. I often just ordered snacks such as fruit and avoided the cooked meals that the hospital offered, as I wasn't fond of hospital food. I'd go on to pass the next few hours watching daytime TV and sitting on my computer until my gourmet Lebanese food arrived. I didn't care that there was a wait because it was worth it. Mum called after my meal to check in, and I couldn't be happier to have finally eaten a quality meal after the days of mass-produced, cold, hospital food. Having to eat the hospital food so often really made me appreciate how good my life was. Really, my entire cancer experience made me appreciate life more as I came to realise how lucky I was to be healthy.

After this, the boredom of being alone really started to kick in so I pulled up my contacts and went to my 'recents' where I saw my cousin

Sebastian - The COVID Holiday

Julian's name. When you're in isolation with only the nurses and doctors in the hospital for company, you become eager to connect with family and friends, and what better way to do that than to call Julian? I ended up speaking to him for ages, just happy to not be stuck with my own company for an hour or so. This was until my mum's voice filled the room yet again when she called the room and the phone automatically answered so that she could say goodnight. I must say that the thought of unplugging the phone really crossed my mind at that moment.

Brushing my teeth was no easy feat with my IV machine which had been pumping saline into me. It was originally pumping antibiotics into my port until we were sure that my symptoms were from COVID and I didn't also have a bacterial infection. Now it was just pumping pure saline which meant that I was lugging around the IV machine like a crippled old man for no good reason but to stay hydrated, as if I couldn't just drink some extra fluids myself. To get to my room's bathroom, I first had to unplug the machine from the wall. Then I turned in circles around the room trying to untangle the cords wrapped around me. After this, I could move to the other side of the hospital room step by step to my toiletry bag, before going back over to the bathroom, brushing my teeth, and doing it all over again in reverse. Timothy and I (Timothy being the name I gave to the IV machine by the way) would spend lots of time together over my treatment as we navigated our way around the many rooms in the hospital. As weird as it may seem, the sight of an IV machine to this day is a nostalgic experience that serves as a reminder of the countless fun hospital experiences I had over my journey through

The ~~Worst~~ Best Year

cancer. Whenever I was staying overnight in the hospital or receiving chemo treatment, I would have Timmy by my side, and I could always count on his beeping to continue no matter what was happening.

I ended up leaving the hospital later the following day, after I had taken a couple of doses of Paxlovid, and my symptoms began to subside. My stay in the hospital was only for a couple of days, but nevertheless, it was very memorable. I soon received the all-clear from Dr Cooper on his rounds to return home. Mum told me she was on her way, and I thought I should start packing my stuff up so I was ready for when she came. My mum was keen to take me back home when she arrived at the hospital and so off we went towards the car park through the staff entrance, accompanied by the nurse in charge. To leave my negative pressure room, we went through a special entry room that had all the equipment the nurses needed before entering my room. On our way out through this side room, I could see Mum eyeing out a small medical box on the shelf just by the doorway. Inside was a stack of orange N95 masks with a wide mouth shaped like a duckbill for extra protection. Before we could leave, she made sure to not miss out on grabbing a couple of the masks to add to her ever-growing stockpile. She couldn't help herself!

"Mum, we have enough at home! Why are you getting more?" I kept my voice to a hard whisper so as to not attract too much attention from the nurse in charge. "Shh Sebastian, we need them".

We didn't really need them, but she couldn't resist the free masks. They weren't cheap either. N95 masks would sell for $2.00 each, so when both of us were going through one a day on each hospital trip and every day I left the house, the ostensibly small cost became quite noticeable. I was also irritated by the fact that Mum chose the wide mother-duck-bill-shaped masks that look as repugnant as wearing a literal duck on your face. In comparison, the other N95 masks were a shade of green that could blend in with a set of scrubs and give a professional look as if I was an actual doctor. I mean, if you're going to take the masks, at least take the good ones. Like seriously!

At home, I went straight up to the isolation chamber, where I would reside until my seven days of isolation were over (that was the government-set isolation period at the time). The next few days involved relaxing at home, where I was free to get some schoolwork done as soon as residual COVID symptoms went away and I had no more excuses to hold me back from doing work. The Paxlovid had kicked in within a day or two. In the space of 36 hours, I had gone from vigorously shivering up a temperature of 39.5°C to barely feeling sick whatsoever. Now this may have been my immune system finally kicking in, although I like to think that the Paxlovid had at least a little to do with it. I was able to achieve more, as my head was no longer so heavy from the high temperatures. When mealtime came around, a food tray would be dropped at my door as per the infamous *Khoury Protocols*. I would wait for my parents to leave, and then I would pick it up to eat, before putting any rubbish in my temporary bin which had been put by my doorway. Since the risk and danger of transmission were low given the precautions we were taking and the fact that Jerome had just had COVID, while Elijah had it a few months prior, there wasn't too much to worry about regarding others becoming sick. In the past when someone had COVID, the whole family would be worried about getting sick, particularly when the strains were more severe and everyone was trying to protect me.

Coming out of my isolation period was a relief, however, I wasn't done with the side effects of COVID yet. The RCH treated you as a COVID-positive patient if you had tested positive within three weeks, even though the government only had a seven-day rule at the time. For the next two weeks of treatment, I would be taking the same precautions that I went through when I was actually sick, which proved to be a silent blessing. The hospital would continue to isolate me from everyone else. Therefore, I would have a private room for all my chemo treatment which could bring some quiet to what would normally be a noisy chemo session with screaming kids in the background.

We had a chemo cycle review coming up with Claira and I would be in the Dolphin Ward. We were told this ward was better equipped to handle infectious disease patients, which may have sounded comforting, but only stressed my mum out about contracting COVID herself. She was worried that since it housed many infectious patients, she would become infected with COVID. Only a week earlier, she was happy to be within a few metres of me without so much as a mask, yet now she was concerned with catching COVID in a ward that had pressurised rooms, and where the only people she was coming into contact with had full PPE gear! The wait to see Claira was long. We had an afternoon

Sebastian - The COVID Holiday

appointment which meant there was plenty of time for delays in her schedule to accumulate throughout the day. At least we had a TV and phones to help us to pass the time.

When Claira eventually came in, she made her way through a checklist of questions to track my recovery from the prior round of chemo treatment whilst also making sure I had recovered from COVID before allowing me to start the next round of treatment. The whole time spent with Claira was no longer than half an hour, yet we spent a couple of hours in the hospital just waiting around. This was frustrating since so much time was wasted from our day, not to mention parking and the 50 minutes spent on the road as we navigated through the city traffic. Now that I was bald, I could see the skin on the top of my head for the first time which meant that a couple of sunspots had become visible. We thought to get the two or three spots checked by Claira on her way out, since we would never really be able to tell if they changed in shape and size after treatment when my hair regrew.

Over the next few weeks, I would have my chemo treatment in the negative pressure rooms on the in-patient ward so that I wouldn't expose any of the cancer patients to the remnants of COVID that may have been lingering. My dad was busy with work for one of my next chemo sessions, and Mum also had an unavoidable commitment, so my uncle George took me. Dad was able to drop me off at the hospital, and Uncle George would then stay with me during the chemo session before taking me home. The only problem with trying to meet up with him in a car park is that there's no phone reception, so while we had

The ~~Worst~~ Best Year

told my uncle which elevator to meet us at, there were many different elevators so it could easily be confusing trying to locate it. Since we were in the car park, communication was limited, and we couldn't call him when we parked. Eventually, after 15 minutes of waiting around, as my uncle was trying to find a car spot, we were able to find him. Just like when I came in to be treated for COVID, we masked up in N95s and called the nurse in charge to take us through the back entrance to the negative pressure room. Since there were strict limits on visitors, I hadn't really had anyone outside my immediate family see me in the hospital yet, making it feel different walking through the hospital with my uncle.

The negative pressure room was the same as the day prior, just how I left it. The 250mL water bottle I had left there the previous day was still there, in the same place. It looked like the room was reserved for me for the week. I had brought some homework with me as it was a school day, and I still had work to complete at 3:00 in the afternoon, which was the time of my chemo session. I was doing some business management schoolwork, taking notes on the benefits and limitations of buying an existing business or starting a new one. The content was quite straightforward, mostly based on common sense. This made for a relaxing chemo session that didn't involve excessive amounts of thinking, unlike the session when I was completing maths methods and was ready to throw the book out of the window. My uncle looked quite relaxed sitting in the cushioned area, and everything was calm. I was getting work done, getting through treatment, and I was in a peaceful mental state. On top of this, it was a short chemotherapy session, meaning that we were zipping in and out of the hospital within two hours, which kept my spirits high and didn't feel too draining. Despite the horrible effects of both COVID and cancer, I was still moving forward.

Chapter 15

Cancer Changes More Than Looks

~ Natalie ~

Our looks were not the only thing that changed. The way people looked at us changed too. It was that look of pity that I came to detest. I was that person with cancer. Sebastian became that child with cancer. When I was introduced, I was Natalie. When I walked away, I sensed their sympathetic whispers: "She's the one with cancer." I felt the same way when Sebastian was sick. Sometimes I wanted to comment out of annoyance, but I always stopped myself. I would pretend that those moments where people looked at you with sympathy never happened. When your hair begins to thin out and your brows follow the same process, it becomes obvious that you have cancer. I hated that cancer defined our lives. My treatment started over the festive season, and I recall people asking me to sit down as they didn't want me to tire myself. This came from a place of care and I have always liked being treated like a princess, but this became frustrating as I thought I must look so sick. I was self-conscious about how I looked. I know everyone had my best interest at heart; however, it was just how I felt at the time. I preferred it when people just treated me as they usually would.

On many occasions, people were unsure of what to say to me. Some avoided me altogether. There is a term called 'cancer ghosting' and this is a real thing. Some people may feel guilty, knowing they fit into this category. This is not my intention. I understand people do not know what to say when confronted with difficult situations, but the avoidance hurt. It was either radio silence from some or too many questions from others.

But what is a happy balance? One question that should never be asked is, "What is the staging?" Rather, this information should be offered by the patient. This bothered me more with Sebastian's diagnosis. My child had cancer regardless of the stage. The fact that my child had been diagnosed with cancer was the most devastating experience of my life and having to verbalise the stage that the cancer had progressed to made me feel sick. The fact that people would ask upset me, resulting in me letting my phone ring out. When these questions were asked in a text, I would ignore the question and thank them for reaching out. People did not mean to be insensitive; they did not understand how I felt. Thankfully, most people have not had to deal with such an experience, so half the time, they are unsure what to do or say. People often now ask me for advice regarding friends of theirs who have been diagnosed with cancer and what they could do to support them. I hate answering these questions as I am not an expert and I experience so much pressure when confronted with questions like these, feeling the need to offer the right advice. I can only tell you what helped us.

On the flip side, though, through both our cancer obstacles, I have developed lifelong friendships, so much so that I call these people family. I enjoyed being in the company of people who I loved. We were surrounded by many generous people who invested their time and energy into cooking meals for us. It meant I had one less meal to worry about cooking and the freezer overflowed with delicious meals. (I would never request an order, although when a beef lasagna with bechamel sauce was delivered, that was an excellent night.) On one particular day, I arrived home from my chemotherapy treatment and my mother-in-law, who was looking after the boys, told me there was a note on the bench from the lady who lived in the weatherboard house across the road. I thought it was strange, as I hadn't even met the lady across the road from us. She was a new parent at our primary school and had heard that I was unwell. She had prepared meals for my family and left me a note introducing herself. This is kindness at its finest. When we received texts from loved ones with messages of support, that gave us strength and kept us going. I appreciated it when people offered to take my children out of the house for a short while. When I was diagnosed my children were so young. It made me so happy when I saw the joy on their little faces when friends organised to take them out for a play or an outing. It also allowed me to get some rest while the children were kept busy. It was a nice change for them as they often saw their mum with her head in a bucket.

A mother's guilt is harrowing. When Sebastian was sick, people kept my youngest son Elijah distracted which was always gratefully welcomed. It hurt that I was unable to be present enough and I felt like I was neglecting my entire family. My entire focus was on Sebastian and his treatment. When I found some free time for myself, it usually consisted of sleeping or crying, and in those moments when I was on my own, I could release the anger and frustration within me. The guilt was eating away at me, as I felt I had neglected my other two children, my husband, my house and my job. I thank God daily that I had George beside me to hold everyone and everything together. It was not easy for George either. He had a job that required a lot of his time and commitment, and he also continued to work and found time for our family. He cooked dinners, cleaned, and did the washing.

Every year, my dear friend Mercy and I would go to Queensland to visit our friend Bec for a girls' weekend. Our trip was organised before Sebastian's diagnosis, booked months in advance. Once Sebastian was diagnosed, I told George to cancel my flight as I wasn't going. George said, "Absolutely not!" I was burnt out by the end of cycle one of Sebastian's chemotherapy and George knew that the trip was exactly what I needed. George spoke to Mercy and together they ensured the trip went ahead. My logical mind at the time knew that I needed this. We were only five days into cycle two, and I was exhausted. We still had ten rounds of cycle two and four more cycles to go. The emotions of the past couple of months were taking a toll and there was still a

The ~~Worst~~ Best Year

long road ahead.

Logically I knew I needed this but my mother's guilt was in overdrive. I was worried about what people would think if they heard I had gone away and left my sick son home with his father. If my friend was in the same situation and had asked for my advice, I would have said, "Who gives a shit what people say? Are they living your nightmare right now?" But in that moment, I was the one battling with those thoughts. I felt guilty about leaving my son while he underwent chemotherapy treatment. Sebastian convinced me to go as I would only miss one chemotherapy session. Sebastian told me he wanted George, his Godfather, to take him. They had a special bond, and time away from me in hindsight was what Sebastian needed at that time. I was so glad that I went. Although I spent most of that time away crying, I was able to do it without worrying about my children seeing me cry. There were also moments of laughter, and lots of wine. The girls were supportive and gave me the fuel to return home energised.

Coming out of this obstacle people ask if cancer has changed me. Of course it has changed me! It has changed me, for the better and dare I admit, for the worse. I used to be more empathetic. If someone was diagnosed with cancer or sick, I would cry. I am still sad to receive sad news, but not as emotional. I feel like I have used up all my tears. But I have also become less trivial. I used to stress about the little things, like a fresh scratch on my new car, but these things are no longer important. They are superficial. My friendships have changed too. I used to put so much energy and effort into anyone who entered my life, but now I appreciate the saying 'quality over quantity'. In one of my counselling sessions, I discovered that I can be passive-aggressive. I used to let things happen even if they upset me, but I exploded when it became too much. Through these sessions I have become more assertive. I am now better at saying what I want and don't want.

Chapter 16

Sickness And Transfusions

~ *Sebastian* ~

I could run, but I couldn't hide from sickness, especially when my immune system was as useless as me trying to stop dozens of doughnuts being dropped off at my door every morning. Don't get me wrong, I really appreciated everyone who sent me doughnuts, but I got over it after the first 20 dozen showed up at my door. I would constantly contemplate whether or not I should see people and go out into the world. Having a social life during my recovery was almost as mentally challenging as recovery itself. Staying home locked away in my room while the rest of the world went on without me was monumentally more challenging on the mind than shivering over a hospital bed on potent antibiotics in peril. So I chose to see people. I couldn't continue being locked away in my room and let my world continue without me.

I obviously took some precautions that one with a struggling immune system might take. I wore an N95 mask where I could and kept a sanitiser on my person at all times, a sentiment I largely follow today. Unfortunately, although sanitisers can be effective, they were no match for the innumerable pathogens crawling in each and every crevasse of the school grounds. As a result, time after time, I would find myself being rushed through the doors of the Emergency Department at the RCH that were all too familiar. Driving there was no small feat. As the parking complex was limited in capacity, Mum and I would often spend half our journey driving laps around the lot. The first time I went into the Emergency Department, I was shivering non-stop, my body shaking uncontrollably. The winding turns of the parking lot added to my discomfort.

After two months of treatment, our trips to the emergency ward had become quite frequent, to the point that it was almost a routine. After scavenging the overcrowded car park for a spot, we would approach the department's reception desk. Before we could, we had to go through a vestibule with security at a makeshift desk with boxes of masks and hand sanitiser to ensure we were COVID-safe. However, in my sickened state, something about going up to the security guard felt rather COVID-unsafe, so I would stay behind in the doorway at a safe distance. The adult masks were the stock standard disposable blue ones, while the kid masks had small elephant patterns on their exterior, luckily way too small for me.

The reception, like many places in the hospital, was often understaffed and so the receptionist was always on the phone with someone when we walked in. The reception area had row upon row of chairs, and only half a dozen were usually filled at one time. I would wait in a secluded part of the waiting room to minimise others' exposure to any pathogens I was carrying and protect myself from theirs, so I found the chair most distant from everyone else and sat there while Mum spoke to the receptionist. Mum told them that I was "Sebastian from the oncology ward", who had yet again spiked a temperature. After speaking such magic words, a door was unlocked, and we were directed straight through to a separate waiting room away from the other sick people. Then the nurses came through and questioned me about my symptoms, from their onset to their recent progression, while taking observations, 'obs' for my heart rate, blood pressure, temperature, you get the jist. It was often a while before another nurse came to move us out of the room as they waited to find space to fit me into the hospital, which was under constant stress and always reaching capacity.

The hospital was particularly busy on this day, and they were struggling. I had my phone charged to keep me busy for the moment, but that could only last so long before the inevitable boredom kicked in. Periodically, a nurse would come in and let us know that they were moving through patients as quickly as they could. It felt as though we were at a restaurant waiting for our food on a busy Saturday night and the nurse was a waiter who had to keep apologising for the delays on our food. Eventually, probably to free up the observation room we were in, Mum and I were moved to a new section (moving tables in the restaurant, if you will). Since I had a respiratory disease, which I could have picked up from anywhere due to my low immunity, I would often be placed in the negative pressure room in the triage section, like when I had COVID. Sometimes I was moved to a standard private room. I just wasn't allowed to be in the hallway interacting with others. Since the hospital was under immense stress and none of these rooms were available that day, the nurse leading us started looking for any closed-off area to put me in. It was on the opposite side of the triage station, next to the negative pressure room, that she found an old supply room. "Are you guys okay if we leave you here until we find a room for you?" she asked. "That's okay, thank you," we replied.

It wasn't glamorous, but at least we were slowly moving through the processing system to finally be treated. The room was packed with Christmas decorations and supply boxes that had accumulated a film of dust. It was the middle of the year, and I was surrounded by Christmas baubles and one of those cheap, tiny, one-metre-high Christmas trees that could fit no more than a metre of tinsel wrapping. There were piles of random storage items and a couple of seats to sit and wait on. Surprisingly, there were many things to explore throughout the room. We left most of the boxes untouched as they were see-through, and you could get a decent clue as to what most of them contained just by looking at them. The nurse told us that she would try to get back soon to get me hooked up to begin treatment but it would take some time, given how many people were in the hospital.

Without hesitation, Mum picked up the phone and called all her friends to tell them we were stuck in a storage room, as if we had booked a hotel for the night and should expect better. I don't know why

The ~~Worst~~ Best Year

"George, they've moved us from the room with two chairs and a desk to the room with two chairs and a Santa Claus," was such an important call but it did pass the time. As for me, I just waited. It was clear that we would be stuck here for a little while, so I didn't call anyone straight away. Looking at things on my phone could only keep me occupied for so long though, and I decided to call my cousin Julian to pass the time. I seemed to do that a lot when I was bored during treatment.

"Hey Jules, guess where I am?"

"Not sure. Where?"

"I am at the hospital."

"Oh, are you okay?"

"Yeah, but they've stuck us in the storage room of the Emergency Department, and I'm bored out of mind." (Now I was the one complaining about being stuck in a room with Santa Claus.)

"Hey, Sebastian!"

His family were in the background, so I thought I'd best give them the tour of my hospital room. "So, pretty much I've got a bed of boxes in the corner over here, some hospital name tags in the boxes over here, and Santa is staring at us over there." This continued for a while until we worked our way over to a closet next to the chair I was sitting on. Given that there wasn't much to do in this boring old storage room, I found some entertainment in opening the old metal closet to my left. To my surprise, there were donations of toys and other items from charity organisations on each shelf. Buried under the pile of toys was a box of muesli bars on the second shelf from the bottom. "Take one,

Sebastian - Sickness and Transfusions

take one!" Julian and his sisters, Martine and Domenique, dared me. Since we weren't exactly getting our dinner meal from the hospital, I thought I was entitled to the muesli bar, so I took one and made sure to get a spare one to give to them. After half an hour of waiting, Mum started to grow wearisome and stated that the hospital staff must have forgotten about us. Given that this room seemed to have been forgotten about since the previous Christmas, the assumption didn't seem so far-fetched.

Not too long after that, a nurse came in with a cart with the equipment needed to access my port. These carts contained half a dozen vertically stacked trays and a bench to work on. Essentially, it was a mobile treatment station stacked with medical supplies. The process would start with the nurse obtaining all the equipment that was needed. From gloves, disposable trays, and alcohol swabs to tweezers for the cotton swabs to clean the port site, bandages and wound coverings, there was a lot to assemble. The nurse would open up the trays one by one and take out the items needed before opening up the surgical glove package and putting them on. Once this happened, they couldn't reopen the cart trays if they'd forgotten something due to the risk of contaminating their gloves, which added to the complexity of accessing the port. I pulled up my jumper so the nurse could put the needle into my port, which was located under the skin on the side of my chest. On the inside, I was a boiling pot as I began to spike a fever, yet a cold shiver ran through my body, and my now exposed skin felt as though it had been covered in a layer of crushed ice.

The ~~Worst~~ Best Year

The needle used to access a port was longer than a typical blood draw needle, and it was L-shaped to stay in position more easily. Early on in my treatment, I would be given Emla numbing cream half an hour before my port was accessed to help with the pain of pushing the long needle into it. I started to get sick of this so I would go on to ask the nurses to put the needle straight in to save time. Given some of the pain you endure when you have chemo, the insertion of a needle like this didn't hurt too much more than a normal blood test. If only I had worked this out sooner, I could've saved a lot of time when accessing my port. The nurse poured alcohol into the plastic disposable tray and soaked some cotton balls in them like chips in tomato sauce. The nurses called this something along the lines of 'the three cleans'. Using the tweezers, alcohol-infused cotton balls would be rubbed in circles around my port to clean the site. It was relieving to have the cool alcohol pressed on my skin with my elevated temperature. Next, she would grab the small protruding lump under my skin; this was my port. "Do you want to look away, Sebastian?"

"No, he likes to watch," Mum would reply. I did like to watch, finding the procedural elements fascinating and orderly. With a count of three, I was pricked as the needle broke the surface of my skin. With a steady hand, the nurse would hold the needle in position whilst grabbing gauze to place in the gap between the needle and the surface of my skin, supporting it in position. This was then covered by a large piece of plastic that held the needle in position before she placed two strips of rectangular stickers where the cords attached to the port ran down the side of my chest. The nurse used some saline and pushed it through the cords of my port, then I felt a quick flush before a few samples of blood were drawn. These would be rushed over to the lab for testing, where they would check the full blood count and blood cultures to detect the presence of any pathogens.

The nurse would soon be back to administer some precautionary antibiotics. Whenever I arrived at the emergency ward with signs of respiratory illness, even when I had tested positive for a virus such as COVID, I was given some broad-spectrum antibiotics in case I was also infected by bacteria. As the tests were yet to return, these measures had to stay in place until my condition had improved. This would be considered over the top for most people with a 38°C temperature, but given my immunocompromised state, once a temperature had reached this level, all precautions were necessary to prevent further illnesses that my body may not have been able to handle on its own.

The nurse promptly returned with a bag of piperacillin-tazobactam, or 'pip-taz' for short. This was the go-to antibiotic whenever I came into the hospital with a potential disease. After being hooked to the IV machine and connected to the cords running out of my port, I would have the pip-taz intravenously every six hours. This was particularly annoying since it meant that I would have my next dose in the early hours of the morning. For now, I had to go to the toilet and it wasn't like the storeroom had its own built-in toilet. The problem was that I was sick and trying to minimise my interactions in the corridors and spaces that other people had access to. I asked Mum what she thought

The ~~Worst~~ Best Year

I should do. "Just go!" Mum didn't seem too worried about me making others sick, so I went up and opened the doorway to the triage desk outside the storeroom. I stood in the doorway so that I maintained a safe distance from the other nurses, patiently waiting to visually make eye contact with one of them to get their attention. However, given how busy the department was and the N95 mask covering most of my face, it was not easy to get the attention of the nurse using facial cues, so I looked over at the nurse manning the triage desk and said, "Excuse me". It took a second, but the nurse looked back. "Would it be possible for me to use the bathroom?"

"Yep, it's just down the hallway on your right." Surprising! I didn't think I would be allowed to use the same bathroom as everyone else when I was sick, but apparently, it didn't concern them too much. I am not sure if the nurse realised that I was sick with a respiratory disease or not, given how busy they were, but I wasn't complaining.

Tugging the IV machine around the Emergency Department was no picnic though. As I was walking towards the bathroom, I kept having to stop every few seconds. The wheels kept locking, the machine would get twisted, and I would have to turn in circles around it to untangle the cords running out from my port connected to the IV machine. I eventually worked out that if I put more pressure on the machine while I walked, it would prevent me from losing control of the wheels. So I didn't have to do the tango with Timmy through the corridor of the Emergency Department as I danced circles around him, trying to get unstuck. The hallway was a sound-chamber of kids screaming in pain, buzzers going off, and doctors scrambling to help different patients. It was a thrilling nightmare; I loved it. Thinking about the rush that the doctors must have had moving from patient to patient, with no room for boredom, brought me back to a time when I was working an understaffed Friday or Saturday night at the pizza shop.

I returned to the room as quickly as possible as I felt so guilty about potentially exposing the people in my vicinity to my sickness despite wearing an N95 mask. Mum was journalling throughout the night in her pink book. What originally was a place where her questions to ask Quinn and Claira were written ended up doubling as a journal, which I dubbed the 'Cancer Bible'. It contained a collection of stories that progressed through her experiences with my cancer and how it transformed our lives. In essence, the pink journal was the first draft of her part of this book. I continued to wonder what she was writing about but never read it. Was it about me? Was she just angry with the world and wanted to make sure that she documented everything? The answer she gave was that she always regretted never journalling when she was sick, and this was her second chance to do it. The memories, like being stuck in a hospital storeroom, are ones that you want to keep for life and journalling them helps to keep them safe.

Later into the night, the nurse came back in with some news. They had called the cancer ward and we were being admitted into a room. Given my sickness, I was wheeled up in a bed while Mum carried our belongings, and a nurse pushed the IV machine. When we arrived at the room, the nurse allowed me out of bed so I could move into the hospital room. After getting ready for bed, I noticed my saline was being pushed through at 100mLs an hour, and I was using the toilet so much that my urine had turned clear, so I asked if it could be reduced. I was drinking water, especially when I took tablets of medication as well. The nurse came and slowed it down a little, although there was still lots of saline coming through. I know 100mLs might not sound like much when stretched over one hour, but when you go to sleep, your bladder fills up multiple times per night. That night, I had a dream that I needed to go to the toilet, where I almost began urinating in my dream-state toilet only to suddenly wake up about to piss myself in real life. My bladder was overflowing with liquid from all the saline that was being pumped through me. A quick check and thankfully, there wasn't any damage. My phone told me it was nearing 6:00 am so no one was up except the night nurse. Unhooking the IV machine, I went over to the toilet in my hospital room as quickly as I could to release my bladder. On the way out of the toilet, since I had already been awoken, I got changed and ready for the day.

When my port was accessed, I only had a shower every second day due to the absurd complexity of taking a shower without getting the port wet. When I wanted a shower in the hospital, the nurse would be called to unplug the cords of my port from the IV machine. My port, draped in needles and short cords, wasn't yet de-accessed as I was still an in-patient in the hospital. Having the port still accessed meant that on weeks I had five days of chemo in a row or when I was in the hospital for a sickness, I would have half showers. There was always

Sebastian - Sickness and Transfusions

a pair of thongs in the go-bag we had packed so that I could have hospital showers without risking warts and other diseases. To not have the needle and port site wet, I invented what I call the shower dance. Essentially, it was the Hokey Pokey. You put your right arm in, you take your right arm out, you put your left arm in, and so on, carefully trying to not wet the right side of my chest. The process was not comfortable, but at least it kept the water bill lower since I really didn't want to spend too long doing a children's dance if I didn't have to.

By the time daylight broke, my illness already seemed to have peeked and I was on the mend. I needed to stay on the pip-taz for the following 36 hours as a precaution. When my blood cultures came back clear of any common bacterial pathogens and my symptoms had subsided, I was cleared to return home after a three-day trip to the hospital. As for the other effects of chemo, the symptoms that stemmed from a low blood count were still not due for another week which meant that for the interim, I could relax.

It was Friday night, time to hang out at Aunty Monique's house. The issue with having plans to do things when your life is so unpredictable is that the plans may change, and adaptability becomes a part of the illness. Over the last few days, I had begun to struggle to move around the house without my heart starting to beat faster than most people's would during a horror movie. After entering the house, I greeted everyone and sat down immediately in the dining room. My heart was beating through my chest, and I could count its beats without even touching it. A glance at the heart rate app on my Apple Watch told me

The ~~Worst~~ Best Year

that I was sitting at 125 bpm, and that was just moving from the car outside to the kitchen table. My parents originally bought the Apple Watch to track my heart rate a year prior when I was having chest pains after my COVID vaccine and once again, its heart-tracking abilities had come in handy. "What are you at?" Mum would constantly ask, her go-to question when she felt the need to check in with me. I usually just read what the watch said and knocked off 10 beats per minute so she didn't worry, until I was sufficiently worried enough to warrant a trip to the hospital. "115." "Do you think we should go to the hospital?" Since I was in favour of delaying the trips until I needed to, I told Mum that I would let her know when we needed to go, and we would probably be good until Monday.

Returning home that night, I recall walking straight up the stairs to my room. I collapsed on the soft quilts of my bed in relief as my heart caught up from all the stairs I had just put it through. My heart was once again jumping out of my chest. As for my head, it was thumping too as my heart worked overtime with a dwindling supply of blood. I didn't want to spend the rest of the weekend lying around in bed with headaches and dizzy spells every time I walked up and down the stairs, but a hospital trip was about as appealing as another night with my head in the toilet. I thought that I'd better check my resting heart rate. Since I had to wait until enough time had passed for my heart to calm down, I spent the next little while scrolling through Netflix trying to find a good show to start watching, to no avail. At this point, I opened the app on my watch back up and loaded the current heart rate. The bottom of the screen read that it was 90 bpm just five minutes prior, although the intense waiting for the number to present itself sent my heart rate flying. It read 97 at first. Then I was nervous about this reading, and it increased to 103 beats and topped out at about 110 bpm. Of course, I wasn't going to worry Mum with that because it wasn't really my resting heart rate anyway, but a nervous one.

Surely enough, when Monday rolled around, I opened my eyes to a pounding in my head despite the fact that I wasn't moving. A quick check of my last recorded resting heart rate at 105 bpm told me it was time to visit our dear friends at the RCH. I told Mum to call and let them know we were coming over for a visit. Dad packed the go bag in the car and I added my computer and toiletry bag. Chemotherapy is good at killing cells, particularly those which can rapidly divide. Purple nails and loss of hair are the visible and trivial unwanted effects of this. However, fertility and bone marrow are also impaired for the same reasons. For me, this meant having a reduced ability to make my own blood cells, leaving me susceptible to infection, and an impaired ability to form blood clots. I also struggled to pump enough blood around my body to carry oxygen to where it was needed, causing my heart rate to rise and extreme headaches. The hospital needed to give me a blood transfusion which would help reverse the symptoms and keep me healthy.

The drive over felt like we were travelling to work. The routine drive from our house to the hospital was a common occurrence, deeply embedded in our memory. Our regular trips to the hospital weren't special or even overly concerning events anymore, but rather they were akin to saying, "I'm off to the shops". Every few minutes, Mum would ask, "What are you at now?" I didn't see the value in checking every five minutes, so I checked once during the trip when we entered the freeway and it was 100 beats per minute. After that, I just added or took away a few beats and pretended to check each time Mum asked until we had arrived.

The problem with the blood transfusions was the long process that it required to be effectively completed. As we had arrived in the morning, the blood testing site in the oncology ward was open for business. It would close at midday, so if we had come later on, we would have had to make a trip to the other side of the hospital for the test. However, thankfully for us, that wasn't the case. In the interest of time, when we entered the ground floor and checked in, I decided to take the two flights of stairs connecting the ground to the cancer ward rather than the elevator which was placed a 60-metre walk away. I had a funny relationship with stairs in that I could never really resist the chance to run up and down them, even when my body was screaming at me to do otherwise and barely permitted it. I couldn't help it. So when faced with the stairs at the RCH, I started running. My left foot on the first step and then two steps at a time after that.

When I was younger, one of my OCD compulsions involved me always finishing the staircase on my left foot to show that the left was somehow superior to the right which was important to me at the time as someone who wrote with their left hand. I didn't care about that anymore, although out of habit, I still climbed stairs in the same way to begin, with my left foot first taking one step and then alternating feet and moving two steps at a time afterwards. It was quite liberating to climb stairs even though I was limited by my sickness. My freedom didn't last too long though, as I struggled my way to the top. Of course, I couldn't help but check if I maxed a new high score on my heart rate monitoring game on the watch. While I didn't quite make the record books, I landed myself a nice 140 bpm which was impressive given how I had only climbed up roughly about 10 metres worth of stairs. Gasping for air, I gave the receptionist at the cancer clinic my name and birthday before sitting down and waiting for Mum to catch up with me.

It wasn't a very long wait before my name was called. "Do you want a finger prick or a normal test Sebastian?" The finger prick was a weird test that was used on kids where someone would prick the tip of your finger and squeeze it for blood. It was a tedious, time-consuming process meant to make receiving the test less painful, although it didn't make much difference, so I asked for the normal phlebotomy test (blood draw), which was far simpler. You might be wondering why on earth I would be having blood taken out of me when I had a shortage of it, an irony not lost on me, however, the hospital protocol was to check the exact blood level to see how much blood to give me. Blood was in short supply at the time, so it wasn't given if not needed by the patient. The protocol also involved testing my blood type. I already knew myself to be O positive, although the test was still conducted in the very rare chance that I could no longer receive O positive blood.

Apart from the hassle of having to do the blood test, these protocols added lots of extra waiting time to the transfusion process, especially since we had to wait for the tests to come back. The blood tests were indicated with an 'urgent' so that the results could be received as quickly as possible. We could wait downstairs in the cafe to pass the time. Mum still had several coffee vouchers to redeem, so we went to the appropriate place and I purchased a salami bagel. The bagel I ate wasn't big but it was jam-packed with enough meat and other ingredients to fill me up. I slowed my eating down enough to elongate the time spent consuming the bagel so that I wasn't going to get too bored waiting for the tests to return. The headaches and tiredness weren't helping with this though. Sitting down for extended periods was hard enough with normal blood counts, but when my count was as low as it was, the symptoms that accompanied it were no cup of tea. For the half of a week between the onset of the symptoms from my low blood count to me receiving a blood transfusion, I would often be stuck in a constant state of drowsiness with my body being deprived of oxygen.

When the results finally came in, there was no surprise that my blood count was low. How low exactly? That was the basis of a new game I would play where I tried to guess how low my count was. While different countries and institutions may use different scales of blood counting, the one we used indicated a normal blood range to be approximately between 120 and 180 units. I felt like I was sitting at around 65-70. In reality, I was at 60. Usually, a transfusion would not be administered if the level was at 90 or higher and my red blood cell count never reached much above the 90-100 mark during chemo.

Sebastian - Sickness and Transfusions

Today, given how blood-deprived I was, a transfusion was essentially guaranteed. To no one's surprise as well, I was still an O positive blood type and so I was free to receive any O blood type. If the hospital had O positive blood available, I would receive that. However, given how short the blood supply was, there was no remaining O positive so I was going to be receiving O negative blood. I couldn't comprehend how we could completely run out of one blood type, especially where there was a large sample size of donors but I know I was lucky to be receiving the unit of blood that I was. A unit of blood was a couple of hundred mLs and would usually suffice to keep my blood count high enough so it wasn't overly dangerous to my health. Occasionally, I would require more blood and sometimes if there was enough blood available, I would receive more.

    I was not sick at the time, which I often would be when I needed a transfusion given how low my blood count was across the board, leaving me extra susceptible to disease. Because I wasn't sick, I didn't have to stay in the in-patient ward but rather could receive my blood in the chemo section and be out before dinner. The nurse brought the bag of O negative blood and confirmed with me that it wasn't my first transfusion. They ask this question since those who haven't had a transfusion before may be prone to having allergic reactions to the blood, so such patients are monitored more closely to make sure they are not one of those people who react. The transfusion takes over 90 minutes, although certain procedures at the start and end push this to about two hours. For instance, my port needed to be accessed. After this, a multitude of double and triple checks would take place to make sure I was the correct person receiving the correct blood because a mistake could potentially be extremely dangerous. "Can you tell me your name?"

"Sebastian Khoury." I also stated my date of birth as it was customary to give this for additional confirmation of your identity, and especially important for me as there was another Sebastian with a very similar last name on the chemo ward during part of my treatment. The nurse then checked the sheet with my blood type of O positive and matched it to the O negative blood bag. I also made sure to check this myself just to be absolutely sure that all was in order. A second nurse was helping to also oversee this process, going through the checks to ensure that the blood was irradiated for my own safety before hooking me up to the bag through the IV machine. The first 15 minutes of the transfusions were the most dangerous. If I was going to have an adverse reaction to the blood, it would occur during the earlier stages of the transfusion as my body would detect the blood as foreign and try to attack it.

The first time I received a blood transfusion was a bit of an ordeal. The nurses were extra cautious to make sure that I wasn't going to have any reaction to the blood. My heart was pumping fast enough before the transfusion from the low count, so the last thing I needed was a nurse telling me that I may be about to have an allergic reaction. I glanced over to the IV machine and carefully counted the first drops of blood dripping down before entering my port. What started as a few drops of red moving through a small, transparent cylinder turned into a stream of blood working its way from the bag to my chest through the thin plastic tubes that ran into my port. We then waited 15 minutes to see if there was any reaction, as if it was a magic number whereby nothing bad could happen after it. The nurse patiently waited by my side until the time was up to make sure I was okay. We were diligent and checked for rashes around my body or any itching that may have presented (just a bit of déjà vu). After that, the process became less daunting. I could finally just relax and get some work done while the machine did its thing.

It had only been a minute of this transfusion, but looking up at the blood-soaked bag, I thought about the person giving blood to me. The thought of them going to their local blood donation site and sitting in the leather chair while they gave blood, all so I could receive it from another chair in a similar-looking room. I started to think about what kind of person they were. They were just one of seven people who would have donated their blood to me during my treatment. How old were they, what was their ethnicity, were they a man or woman? I genuinely wanted to know about who they were, except I was never going to find out given the confidential nature of blood donation. It was 15 minutes in, and while I wasn't really worried about having an adverse reaction, there was a small internal sigh of relief as the clock ticked over, reassuring me that everything was going to be okay.

We were doing logarithms in maths and were up to the revision stage. Somehow, I had forgotten so much of the content we had covered during the topic, and I felt like there was some ground to make up.

The ~~Worst~~ Best Year

I had completed all the work, yet the revision was tough. Some of the calculations we had to solve without a calculator were extensive, allowing for careless errors to add up. I sat there the entire time going through the same problems until I was thoroughly confident with them.

Chapter 17

Cancer Kills More Than The Body

~ *Sebastian* ~

What do you do when you have cancer? Everyone does what makes sense to them. This will look different for every cancer patient. I continued to focus on the importance of schoolwork and tried to ignore everything that was trivial. I kept my walls high like an emotional fortress and rarely entertained grim ideas. It wasn't until I spoke to my psychologist that I admitted to another person what I was worried about—I was worried about not being me and not performing to the high standard that is expected of me. I must have sat in my psychologist's office for two minutes straight, imbued by silence, just reflecting upon how hard it was going to be for me during treatment. Prior to change, it's difficult to identify what will work best, but prioritising is important. I knew that there would be limitations to what I could possibly manage while undergoing treatment. My body couldn't even manage to run for more than five seconds without becoming puffed. Despite this, I managed to focus on the important tasks, and that allowed me to achieve academic success without overworking myself. However, I did have to lower my standard a little bit.

My mental health suffered throughout my cancer journey. However, it was the love and support of those around me who kept me strong. I was lucky to be surrounded by a supportive community that cared for my every need. It was a regular occurrence for people to pop in for a visit. It helped to keep me sane while the world was going on without me, so I wasn't left out of it. I had former co-workers visiting, along with aunties, uncles, family and friends who I hadn't seen in years. Everyone wanted to offer their support. Even after treatment, some of the people who reached out when I was sick for the first time in a while have managed to continue to stay in touch. My connection with the people who were already close to me prior to my diagnosis and treatment has continued to strengthen, and this closeness will undoubtedly extend beyond my time in the beds of the RCH.

Being in the hospital for long chemo days often felt as slow as shopping with my parents on a Saturday afternoon. During the last four cycles of chemo (each cycle lasted 3-4 weeks, if there were no delays) I would kick things off with an eight, sometimes even ten, hour day of treatment. The morning was filled with hydration which accompanied the cyclophosphamide chemotherapy, and the hydration of liquids alone could last hours. When coupled with my mum checking in on me every so often, I would easily become annoyed. I know that Mum's check-ins were clearly out of love and concern, and I do appreciate her for that.

However, it definitely could get on my nerves sometimes, and so when this happened she would often go for walks to clear her head and give the agitated Sebastian some space. This was our little system so as to not go mad when spending so much time together for six months.

Occasionally, Betty would come in to play a game which was a nice distraction from anything I had going on. Betty came in during the late morning on this particular day. I could see the zipped bag with *Bananagrams* in her hand, and I was excited to play. As this was an eight-hour chemo day, I had a separate room to receive the chemo in, rather than being in a room with many others which was the usual if I was staying for the shorter two-to-three-hour chemo days. This room was one of the rooms used to access my port and was located across the hall from a bathroom and down the hall from the famous chemo bell that patients ring when they have finished treatment. The room had the standard hospital-issued bedside table which was great for *Bananagrams* and was able to fit Betty, my mum and I all in the one space. I was pretty good at the game, relative to Mum at least, so I had my fair share of wins. Although, sometimes I enjoyed losing more so that I could see Mum snap a selfie of the game. I couldn't help but giggle and poke faces in joy, as beating me was some kind of special achievement.

In between each game or two, I was off to the toilet to check whether or not I was hydrated. I hadn't drunk much water and the hydration being pumped into me had only just started, so I knew I wasn't likely to be ready. You were fairly sure after urinating in the

The ~~Worst~~ Best Year

bottle whether you were ready to begin treatment or not, even before the test was run on the sample. I had become quite the expert on the matter. My streams were thin and dark and so it became clear to me that I was not getting chemo anytime soon. So, it was back to the room and drinking away until I was adequately hydrated. Betty was soon off. Mum was too as it was at that point when we had become sick of being in the same room together. She would often go for walks through the hospital and visit the cafe where she could redeem a coffee voucher. This allowed us to have space from one another, as I am a bit of a lone wolf. I like being alone with my thoughts, doing work or just relaxing. Don't get me wrong, I enjoy being in the company of others, but I will often go for long periods just being by myself. That's the way I like it. I had my computer, and I could finally complete some work, which I did.

My window overlooked the wide, spacious green lands around the hospital. In between patches of nature were brightly coloured playgrounds with monkey bars and twirly poles that I had no idea the purpose of. In the mid-afternoon, the clear blue skies were the most peaceful thing my eyes could see, and I was comforted by the warmth of my bed. Many families would walk the concrete track with their extended families and friends, escaping whatever heartache awaited them in the hospital. Inwardly, I dreamed of walking the footpath and being comforted by the *apricity of the sun* shining through the clouds on a winter's morning; unfortunately for me, I was stuck with Timmy for now. Mum had given me around 45 minutes of my own space, and prior to leaving she had asked whether I wanted any food on her way back up. She was at a restaurant located in the corner of the hospital, which was hard to see if you weren't looking for it. She told me they had pizzas, so I asked for a barbeque chicken one. I wouldn't normally ask for a chicken pizza, but I remembered the experience when I worked at the pizza shop, trying all the different ones on the menu, and that the chicken pizza stood out. I didn't mind eating chicken on pizza from time to time if it meant that I wasn't eating the same food over and over again. There were a couple more hours of schoolwork to complete for the day, so getting a start on it made sense.

Timothy was like my child and his beeping was its way of crying and telling me that it needed tending to. As soon as it started beeping, my right arm instinctively snapped straight over to the silence button on the IV machine while my left grabbed the TV remote with the nurse call button. If only I could have muted the children's cries at the RCH with the silence button as well. Since I knew Mum would be on her way, it was time to put my computer away so there was space on my bedside table for the pizza when it arrived. Meanwhile, the nurse had managed to be close by when I pressed the button and quickly changed over the chemo. For those of you wondering about restrictions on food when on chemo, there weren't any. I could eat anything that wasn't going to make me sick, and with the fosaprepitant anti-nausea drug I was given not too long before, I couldn't vomit even if I tried. The drug worked for 72 hours, hence the nickname my mum gave it, 'the 72-hour drug' (as she couldn't pronounce fosaprepitant). Therefore, I could eat what I wanted for lunch without the fear of vomiting as I had on my

The ~~Worst~~ Best Year

first night of chemo.

Betty was one of many tutors in the cancer ward. Occasionally, on the longer chemo days, some of the others would pop in. When they did, Mum would immediately be off to redeem one of her coffee vouchers so I could work with the tutors. While Betty let me take care of my academics on my own, the other tutors who didn't know me that well were a bit different. Instead of playing *Bananagrams*, they would want to complete work with me. While I do have the utmost respect for these people, the questions they would ask me were often targeted far below my academic level and any questions I did have seemed to be a little out of their reach. Which is quite understandable; I was in a children's hospital, after all. Either way, it was still nice to have someone there to talk to every so often even when it did sometimes get on my nerves. Even the nurses and doctors would comment on my schoolwork sometimes and to be honest, I wonder if I brought them back to some less than happy school days.

After the tutor left, Mum hadn't returned, so I was left to complete some maths work. I was working on a non-calculator section of the textbook, which meant my exercise book was filled with line upon line of complicated and intensive work that barely made sense to me. "Beep, Beep, Beep!" Without even noticing, the beeping was silenced, a nurse was called, and I was back to work. When they came in, the nurse commented on the maths work I was doing. "Is that maths methods Sebastian?" she asked.

"Yep, do you miss it?"

"Not one bit. I can barely remember what I learned back then, so I'm probably no use to you."

It soon dawned on me that one day I would probably also come across a kid doing maths methods work, and I would recall the excruciating memories that came with it. One of the challenges when completing my maths work was holding a pen or pencil. As my nails underwent lots of change, I was now left with a dark purple crescent at the base where the nail would normally be white and the nail was now brittle and fragile like a cold chip. This not only made cutting the nails uncomfortable, but I would worry that the nails would snap as they were so brittle. Holding a pen was also a challenge as my left thumbnail would be sensitive if it came into contact with my pen. I think I was worried about them snapping so much that merely touching them with a pen made me uncomfortable. Interestingly, I don't think I made the mental connection at the time, however, I noticed that I took on an Obsessive Compulsive Disorder (OCD) trait which was connected to the fragility of my nails. The physical affliction to my nails was more detrimental in the mind.

I have had OCD for as long as I can remember, and it is constantly manifesting itself through new compulsions or rituals that I feel obliged to complete in an effort to prevent a bad, very unlikely event from happening. In this case, it was likely that the fragility of my fingernails, despite there being no incident where my nails were damaged, made me concerned that I was going to accidentally kick off one of my big toenails when I was walking barefoot around the house. One day

The ~~Worst~~ Best Year

when I was walking barefoot to my room, I was overwhelmed by an unforgiving urge to cover my big toe. What started out as a harmless way of protecting my fragile nails soon turned into a demon inside of me. The demon convinced me that I had to put the toe adjacent to my big toe over the nail when taking a step forward to almost hold it in position so it wouldn't be kicked off. No matter how ridiculous this sounds, resisting the commands of the demon is no small feat. As long as I didn't put myself or someone else in danger, I would listen to it. It had a significant grasp over me, and I was a slave to whatever it told me to think and whatever it told me to do to myself. I know that my actions with OCD often are unreasonable and don't make sense, but the fear of something bad happening makes me think that a few-second ritual of adjusting my toes is worth it, until I'm doing this non-stop, and a few seconds accumulate into much longer.

I had a routine appointment coming up with my psychologist. I would normally do these in person wherever possible. However, with the current circumstances it ended up that my appointment was online. Of course, given the new OCD ritual, I told my psychologist about it. Knowing my psychologist and the treatment we had completed in the past for OCD, I knew exactly how he planned on treating me. The only reason I hadn't started the treatment myself was because the ritual was so new that I hadn't worked up the courage to try it. My treatment for any compulsion often involves challenging the validity of the thoughts I have and in the case of an action-based compulsion, I would attempt exposure therapy, where I am essentially exposing myself to the anxious feeling I had when walking barefoot around the house without enacting the compulsion. The psychologist said to me, "You probably already know what I'm going to say".

"My shoes are already off," I replied with a light giggle. I spent the next little while walking up and down the house without covering my big toe with another toe. As my OCD is often less problematic in the presence of other people, I was able to quickly become accustomed to the anxious feeling of not covering my big toe when walking in the presence of my psychologist. Then when I would later walk by myself, I was able to resist the temptation to cover my toe.

It seems obvious: you beat OCD by just not giving in to it. Although it's not as simple as telling someone who has OCD to just not have it, when someone can confront stressful stimuli in a safe environment, desensitisation to it becomes a possibility. It's by no means easy, and to this day, I struggle with compulsions that are infinitely more complex and burdensome than ones such as this, but the core principles of what makes me act the way I do and the treatment for overcoming it don't change. There was a whole wide-reaching network of people beyond just my family and friends, including people like Betty and my psychologist, who were responsible for helping me mentally throughout my treatment.

Chapter 18

The Last Chemo

~ Natalie ~

You never know what each day has in store for you. Placing our worries aside is easier said than done. As a result of our experiences, we become conditioned to expect the worst, so we stress about circumstances that may not even occur.

Sebastian went through a lot during his treatment. He was in extreme pain after 15 days and we still had a long road ahead of us. However, he continued to jump over every hurdle that presented itself. After round three of his chemotherapy treatment, Sebastian required his first of many blood transfusions as his haemoglobin levels would drop. Two weeks before the final treatment, Sebastian went into the hospital for a routine blood test. On the way, I told him that I thought he looked good. I didn't think that he would need a blood transfusion on this occasion. Sebastian wasn't so convinced. He replied, "I am 75% sure that I will have a blood transfusion today". He had become so attuned with his body that he was right. We arrived at the hospital, and he not only required a blood transfusion but needed two bags of it. Sebastian always masked how he was feeling so that he would not worry me. Although he did not want to worry me, he also did not ignore his symptoms. He used to monitor his heart rate on his Apple Watch. He would check his blood pressure and temperature to work out when it was time to visit the hospital or if we should wait at home. This action made managing the situation easier because every hospital trip was warranted. Although 'easy' clearly did not define our circumstances.

Although the doctors gave Sebastian the all-clear from cancer after round two of chemotherapy, treatment needed to continue for four more rounds, as cancer cells may have still been present in his body. Not only did he have to complete four more rounds of chemotherapy, but the intensity of the treatment was also increased. This program extended some of our chemotherapy sessions to the duration of eight to ten consecutive hours. The results were astounding when we viewed the scans before treatment and compared them to the scans post-treatment. I now have a newfound respect for Sebastian's affinity towards modern medicine. The same drug that had made him so sick had cured him and made him so well. Viewing the clear scans of all those cancer spots was the most liberating feeling. Even the chemotherapy burn he experienced later that day did not put a damper on our day. However, I also knew he still had such a long road ahead.

August 31st, 2022 was the last day of chemotherapy, and we experienced so many mixed emotions. Sebastian spent the majority of the final rounds of chemotherapy treatment in the hospital with respiratory illnesses and blood transfusions. The final two rounds took a toll on everyone. Sebastian's moods were erratic; sometimes, he was happy and other times down. It was extremely tough when he was at his lowest point as he was so sick and there weren't any words that would help him to feel better. The night before the final chemotherapy session I didn't sleep. I was anxious that chemotherapy would be delayed, and my mind was imagining the worst-case scenarios.

A few days before his last chemotherapy session I was out to breakfast with my cousin Carol from Sydney. Although Carol lived in a different state, she always supported me through phone conversations. I was apprehensive about heading out with her, as this was during the COVID period. I mostly kept a very low profile throughout Sebastian's treatment, trying to avoid bringing home any viruses that could affect his immunity and stop him from receiving his treatment. When I did go out, I was very compulsive with hand hygiene and avoided kissing people when greeting them. Carol wasn't always in Melbourne, and I didn't want to miss out on the opportunity of seeing her.

At breakfast I bumped into someone I knew, and she kissed me hello before I could pull back. She confirmed that she was not feeling well; her runny nose was very obvious. This caused frustration as people did not realise how immunocompromised chemotherapy patients are and the risks they face when they become sick. The hypochondriac in me took over, and I spent the next couple of days worrying about becoming ill or making Sebastian sick, which would affect completing

Natalie - The Last Chemo

his last treatment on time. I was also worried that if I contracted COVID, I would not be able to attend his last chemotherapy session and hear him ringing that bell. I had heard that bell ring so many times over the six months for other cancer patients. Whenever I did, I would imagine the day that Sebastian would ring it, walking out of those double doors, never looking back. Thank God that day came without any hurdles.

I purchased presents for all the administration staff, nurses, doctors, social workers, teachers and Betty the tutor. I wanted to celebrate and thank everyone for all the support they had provided us over the last six months. Dr Quinn gave us the all-clear to do the final chemotherapy session; we had much to celebrate. We just wanted this ordeal to be over without any delays.

Sebastian's final chemotherapy session was only 15 minutes long, which was a fitting way to end this obstacle. George waited patiently in the waiting area until the chemotherapy was fully administered. As usual, the COVID 'one person rule' did not allow him to come in with us. Once completed, the time had finally arrived for Sebastian to ring the bell. George was allowed to be present for that. Ringing the bell signified the last day of treatment and every cancer patient is given the opportunity to ring the bell, although when I finished treatment, I did not ring the bell. I cannot recall the reason for this. Sebastian had the special job of ringing the bell for both of us. After he rang the bell, I could not miss the opportunity for closure and ring it for myself. The bell ringing is your final farewell from the ward. At the RCH, the cancer patients chose a song to leave to.

The ~~Worst~~ Best Year

All the staff created a guard of honour and lined the corridor. Throughout the six months we were there, I experienced goosebumps each time I heard the sound of the bell. I remember the first time I heard the bell ring. It was during Sebastian's first round of chemo. I was reading Alex Fevola's biography (*Silver Linings: A Journey to Happiness*) and was up to a sad chapter that pulled at my heartstrings. My emotions ran high, and tears flowed freely while I read. I was sad about the chapter that I had just read and sad about being at the hospital watching my son go through chemotherapy. Then, I recall seeing this little girl, about knee height, and she was preparing to ring the bell. The staff called us over to celebrate with her. When she rang the bell everyone started to cheer and her mother broke down and cried. I absolutely lost it. Sebastian was hooked up to the chemotherapy IV while doing his homework. When I returned, he saw me crying and asked, "How old is she, Mum?" I replied that she was only little, maybe three years old. He just smiled and returned to doing his homework, and I returned to reading my book. Reading Alex Fevola's biography enabled me to see that although someone travelled a difficult path, there could also be light at the end of the tunnel. I read a lot of books during Sebastian's treatment. They took me to another place for a short time. I think studying took Sebastian to another place that helped him deal with what was happening to him.

There were many other times I heard the bell ring, and I would cry every time. I pictured this moment in my head each time. The nursing staff would present the cancer patient with a gift to celebrate the end of treatment. Rickey was our nurse on Sebastian's final day of chemotherapy. It was very fitting as Rickey was our favourite nurse. He was there from day one on the ward when Sebastian received chemotherapy for the first time, that not-so-good Good Friday. He was there on Sebastian's last chemotherapy day to unhook him for the last time. God willing, he never has to be hooked up to chemotherapy ever again. Rickey supported Sebastian throughout his entire treatment. The morning was perfect.

Sebastian picked the song *Black Betty* to walk out to. It was an ongoing joke as Betty was his tutor in the hospital, and they spent hours together. She was my lifeline when I was doing so much of this on my own due to the COVID restrictions. As I couldn't work most of the time that Sebastian was sick, George had to continue working to support the rest of the family. He would take the boys to school and after-school activities. Betty would check in on us regularly, and if I needed a break, she would encourage me to take a walk or grab a coffee. She would sit and study with Sebastian or play word games, which he loved. He also loved to beat her. I can recall a long nine-hour chemotherapy day, and Sebastian was a little delirious. He started to play the song *Black Betty* and danced along to it. I was reduced to laughter while watching how he danced. Betty had not come in on that particular day, so he played the song in tribute to her.

A couple of days before we finished chemotherapy, we talked about what song he would walk out to. I suggested that Black Betty was the theme song of his treatment and was fitting to ring the bell to.

The ~~Worst~~ Best Year

The song was perfect as it was an upbeat tune with everyone dancing as he walked out. Betty came down to give him gifts and handed me a bouquet of flowers. The bond we made with the staff at the hospital was so beautiful. Hearing that bell ring was the best sound in the world. Our boy did it! He faced many obstacles, and he conquered stage four Hodgkin lymphoma. His life may never be the same again, but he will find his new normal and achieve great things.

We arrived home, and Jerome was waiting to congratulate him. George, Sebastian and I went out for an ice cream to celebrate. Sebastian received a message from his tennis coach saying, "Okay bludger, when are you getting back to the courts?" Sebastian responded, "See you there tonight". I thought he was joking because he had just finished chemotherapy. Usually, after chemotherapy he would be completely knocked out. Sebastian was running on adrenaline when we arrived home, though. He grabbed his racket and said, "Let's go!" His coach, Jason, was so happy to see him and kept his sunglasses on as he was tearing up the whole time watching him play. Jason was a fantastic support to Sebastian throughout his treatment. He always called and checked in on him. Jason took it slow on Sebastian that afternoon but seeing him back on the court was so good. He built his tennis skills before all this started and had such a passion for the court. It was so lovely to see him return to the courts!

That night, our house was full of friends and family coming to celebrate this wonderful day. There was no plan. It was funny how they all rocked up at the same time. They brought cakes, gifts and

Natalie - The Last Chemo

balloons, making the night a huge celebration. Sebastian was so tired and because of all the excitement, we forgot that he had just finished his sixth round of chemotherapy. He was still running on adrenaline and having the time of his life celebrating with our friends and family. It was a fantastic night celebrating, but he needed to rest.

The last week in August is when the Cancer Council celebrates Daffodil Day. It is a fundraising event that raises money and awareness in the fight against cancer. The daffodil symbolises rebirth and hope. When Sebastian finished treatment, that was exactly how I felt. Sebastian is my hero. August 31, 2022, was the first day *(rebirth)* of the rest of his life, and the day we started our healing once more, the day we found hope. I mentioned earlier that you do not know that you have lived your worst day until you do. You also only know that you have lived your best day once you do. This day was my best and one I thank God for every night before I put my head down to sleep.

Chapter 19

Is The Journey Really Over?

~ *Sebastian* ~

Ring, ring, ring! I forcefully grabbed that bell and shook it in jubilation. The hallway was lined with the medical staff who helped me throughout my cancer journey. By no means were they all there, but the ones who were present symbolised the entire support network that had tirelessly worked together to bring me to health. The joyous walls sang my praises, congratulating me on a journey well done. "I want to ring the bell as well." Mum was just as excited if not more than I was for completing chemo. Mum deserved to ring the bell too. She didn't get to ring any bell that marked the end of her treacherous experience back when she had chemo. After being by my side for the last six months, she'd earned the right to ring it. The bell was a timeless token of hope for those who endured the hardships of chemo, those whose heads were over toilet seats, and bones trembling above their feet. The bell was a symbol of health for those who had surmounted the ultimate fight with cancer. The bell ringing was the supposed pinnacle of a civil war within your body, a war you won.

My proudest day was winning that war. I didn't do anything apart from survive, and survive I did. The nurses handed me gifts with vouchers and warm regards. All that was left to do was to be de-accessed one last time. Rickey ushered me off into the closest room and pulled out the cart with all the medicines. One step at a time, he peeled off the layers of bandage that covered my port until just the needle remained. On his count of three, Rickey yanked the needle, and I was free.

At home, Mum scrolled through social media sites such as Facebook and Instagram. She was looking through all of the heartfelt messages people had sent through to celebrate the end of my chemo treatment. Among them was a message from my tennis coach, jokingly entreating me to come down and have a hit. *Why not?* I thought. Yes, it was true that I could not run for more than three seconds without getting puffed, but nothing could calm my high at that moment except the passing of time, so the only logical thing was to make the most of it while it lasted. Before Mum could finish telling me, I was off to the laundry room where my gear was to grab my racquet and get in the car. The courts were only 800 metres from our house, right by my old primary school, which meant we were there mere minutes later. "Legend! I can't believe you actually came." I don't think he considered when he was joking about me coming down to the courts that he was talking to Sebastian, and Sebastian likes to do crazy things, as anyone who knows me would attest to.

The ~~Worst~~ Best Year

I would usually walk down to the courts myself, or Dad would drive me and return home, except he wasn't going to miss this. I came out on the courts and started to hit some balls. Jason was clearly taking it easy on me, as he should have been, but just the movement on the court made me feel normal again. Unfortunately, Jason was quite fond of the occasional drop shot and didn't shy away from the odd one. The only problem was that since my running capacity was quite limited, I was very hopeless in reaching those. Every so often, I would look over at Dad and see him taking a burst of photos of me striking the ball. I was blessed to be surrounded by people who were happy for me to be back.

Physically, I was just as sick as I had been in every other treatment cycle. I still had the same chemo in me that I had for the last six months, and I still managed to end up back in the hospital in the coming weeks with another risky respiratory disease. I still felt the same tiredness, but I was not going to let that stop me from doing what was important. Physically, I was going to take things easy, but anything that held importance in my life was going to take precedence. The cancer had taken enough away from me. It had taken time away from school, from family, and from friends, and it had stolen time from my life. That night, we had some people over to mark the end of my journey. Cake was eaten, and a bell rung, ringing in the new season of my life.

I soon returned to school. Not just the half days, but fulltime. I was careful about being exposed to others, but less careful; careful about over-exerting myself, but less so. I was even staying back at school again to do homework. One day, a couple of weeks after I returned to school, I was in the library at a private booth, and I started to itch from the bottom of my hamstrings and around my coccyx. Probably nothing, right? While the itch used to be a sign of cancer, the chances of it being back were incredibly low. After all, an itch could be the result of just about anything. So I decided I didn't need to tell anyone. A simple tablet of Telfast that I kept handy from when I used to get frequent itches should do the trick. I took a tablet, and went back to work. However, when my skin erupted in a localised tingling the next day, I was in a bit of a predicament. Was this in my head? Was I manufacturing the itch by thinking about being itchy? The itch began to intensify so much that I couldn't focus on schoolwork. I was in class, so I didn't have my Telfast on me at the time. I figured that I could wait until my return home and take the tablet there.

The itch continued, so I walked up to the office and asked the office receptionist if she could give me Telfast, and they called my mum. As she came over, it hit me: *What if I had cancer again?* I wasn't worried about dying; I wasn't even concerned about how it would affect my body. I didn't want the inconvenience of the situation to return, and I didn't want to be the inconvenience anymore. I was sick of being a burden on my family and if I was sick again, they would be heartbroken. My mum would have to watch me go through treatment again and she would never find peace.

Needless to say, as soon as my mum heard about the possibility of me being sick, we were back to see Quinn in a matter of days. He felt every lymph node there was to feel on the surface of my skin. "Don't worry if any are inflamed, I'll feel them," Quinn said. That probably would have been more comforting if he was able to feel them the first time I was sick but I guess he wanted to reassure us. His conclusion was simple—I was likely experiencing prednisolone withdrawal. It's quite common that some of the symptoms that someone may have experienced in the past may be present when withdrawing from the steroid. It was also really unlikely that the cancer even had time to form given our most recent scans, which were clear. Well, there was at least an alternative explanation, but a scan was needed for clarification.

It wasn't long before I was on the lower ground floor of the hospital at the imaging centre receiving the scan. One of the benefits of the hospital's imaging centre was the outfits that you would wear. Unlike the awkward gowns that were available at the local clinic, the hospital had actual clothes instead of an open gown that you could wear if you needed to change. The nurse went through the standard drill of questions they had to ask, and enquired about all of the potentially metallic objects I may have had on my person. She then handed me a booklet with a list of the movies and TV shows to choose from as entertainment during the scan. Off came my necklace, watch and phone to be handed to Mum before she left. The nurse led me over to a locker to put my shoes and the rest of my belongings in. I punched in my four-digit code and told the nurse to load up the *Big Bang Theory,* season one.

To call the machine loud would be an understatement. Over the many PET and MRI scans I had received throughout my journey, I had started to become accustomed to the deafening banging. However, blocking out the noise completely is never a real possibility. It served as a nice distraction other than the laughs from watching the *Big Bang Theory*. If my mind was occupied by the noise and TV, it wouldn't be thinking about the scan and the results. What if the spot near my coccyx which was metabolically active at my previous scans was actually dangerous and never fully dissipated? It would explain why the itch was primarily in that region of my body.

Thoughts of negativity were as dangerous as the disease itself, and I had to avoid such thoughts at all costs. I had once again gone into survival mode and that meant focusing on life as if everything was normal. The scan was a precaution and a precaution only. I was healthy and the itch could be explained by a million other things. I couldn't put my life on hold every time I was tired and sick, or itchy, because if I did I would never get to live my life. To my surprise, this worked. I was content with whatever happened now. If I was sick, I wasn't going to care about being a burden or missing life. I was going to make the most of another chance to experience something new and see parts of the hospital I hadn't seen before. I didn't want the scans to show anything bad, but I was mentally prepared for it. I didn't tell anyone about these thoughts, figuring that no one would understand the outlook I had. In hindsight, it probably would have been helpful, given how stressful a time this was.

The scan was soon over, and one of the two nurses approached to pull me out. As for what happened next, Mum had a different approach to me—storming through the cancer ward to get the results as soon as possible. The receptionists were busy clicking away on their computers. I always wondered what receptionists were really doing sitting on their computers when there weren't any patients to be processed. Were they just clicking randomly or genuinely busy? Was there data that needed to be inputted? Maybe they were just playing games or checking emails. Whatever emails they were checking were going to have to wait as Mum soon got their attention with a passionate "I need to see Dr Quinn!" My mum was demanding to see Quinn, or at the very least, that he would review the scans as soon as possible and ensure there was nothing out of line. She wasn't going to wait for any exam report or our next appointment. I didn't personally agree with this approach, but if it was going to provide her with the mental peace she required, then I was all for it. It was going to be a wait, but Mum was willing to sleep there overnight if that was what it took. She wasn't leaving without more information.

"You can go downstairs and get some food if you want, I'm waiting here and will call you up when they're ready," Mum said to me. I wasn't keen on food at this point, so the couches in the waiting room were going to do for now. What could I do while waiting for the results that were going to tell us if we were going back to the beginning? I knew that the chances of there being something bad were low, but still seemed high enough for concern. While I had no problem waiting to see my fate, I wasn't sure what to think if I was ill again. I was sick of being sick; I was done with chemo and all that came with it; I was ready to return to normal. Having grown up a lot over the six months, I had learned about the importance of family, and that was great. Nevertheless, having learned what I could from cancer, it had nothing good left to offer me. I had extracted every positive out of living with cancer that I could. The thought of returning to the days of drawing sympathetic eyes every time I walked into a room was almost as daunting as the fear of dragging people down with me for a few more months of chemo. The door to Quinn's office opened, and out came the previous patient. Déjà vu, confusion, excitement, I waited for Dr Quinn to finish off the notes from his last appointment and call us up. Our eyes were fixed on the half-open door. We stared and waited patiently until the magic word "Sebastian" was called and we could enter.

"So, you had the scans. Let's have a look." Quinn opened up my file with all of the notes contained on me as a patient of the RCH. On the top right-hand side was my diagnosis of cancer and the age of diagnosis. Underneath this were notes from all our appointments with Quinn and Claira. Under my scans was my most recent scan. Quinn clicked on the tab, informing us that the in-depth report, which would more conclusively determine whether or not there was anything out of place with the scan, would not be out for a little while longer. Pulling up the document with the scans, Quinn furiously right-clicked and adjusted the imaging to show the relevant parts, dragging on features and scrolling to find the right option to press before analysing it himself. At last, judgement time had come. I could feel my mum's nerves, knowing just how much this meant to my family. "From what I can see, the scans are clear. You don't have anything to worry about." I was relieved, excited,

The ~~Worst~~ Best Year

and liberated. I could now rest easy, knowing that the slight risk that I still had cancer was extinguished. I was now free to live my life; my family was now free from excessively caring for me. Finally, I was excited to press play on living.

Cancer had thrown a spanner into the works of my life. Along the way, I also had the support of an entire community around me. Those who kept me company, who donated their time whether it be taking me to appointments or playing games of *Bananagrams*, all of those who sent doughnuts, no matter how much I dreaded them. You all made cancer a little easier. My friends at school were always there for me and understood my limitations. My family knew how and when to show sympathy and provide me with support. The people I forged connections with during my sickness remain close to me today. My gratitude for their sacrifices makes them key elements of my success.

Chapter 20

So Many Wonderful Charities

~ *Natalie* ~

When you receive a cancer diagnosis, your loved ones rally around you to find ways to lift your spirits. To put a smile on Sebastian's face, we had friends who organised Zoom calls and video messages with Carlton footballers. Sebastian was a passionate Carlton Football Club supporter. Whenever one of these calls was organised, a smile appeared on his face from ear to ear. Our neighbour organised for the Carlton football team to sign a jumper for him, which he absolutely loved. My cousin organised for the team to do a video message to Elijah on his 11th birthday, as it was going to be spent in the hospital with Sebastian on day one of chemo. These acts of kindness made such a significant impact.

When I had cancer, the only two organisations I knew of were the **Cancer Council** and the **Leukaemia Foundation**. These organisations were genuinely supportive and were my go-to for questions and support at a very confusing time. Both these organisations do so much in the way of cancer research. With stats like one in two Australians will be diagnosed with cancer by the age of 85, cancer research is extremely important. When Sebastian was diagnosed, many organisations had a positive impact through his cancer obstacle, for which I will be forever grateful.

One of the organisations we encountered in the early days was **My Room**. My Room is covering the cost of storing Sebastian's fertility until he turns 18. This is wonderful as it was one less thing we needed to worry about.

Redkite gifted us a huge red bag on day one with information, and necessities like grocery vouchers and toiletry essentials—all the basics that came in handy. They also provided the counselling session that I had with other parents, which helped me immensely with the healing process. Redkite offers many services from scholarships to family support. Before Sebastian's diagnosis, I was unaware that this organisation existed, and now I am looking at ways to give back to them.

The Children's Cancer Foundation helped to pay for extra counselling sessions that Sebastian and I benefited from, especially in those early days. They also funded a lady who was located on-site at the Children's Hospital, ensuring that the children and parents had everything they required. This lovely lady used to visit the day chemotherapy ward, distributing treats to parents and children. She was always located in the Kookaburra Ward, where most long-term chemotherapy patients stayed. Sebastian used to hear her voice from down the corridor and waited for the treat he would be given. Her visits provided us with joy. The Children's Cancer Foundation provided me with an ongoing pass to use in the hospital gym so that my mental health was not compromised, as well as giving me time for myself. Going to the gym helped with my back pain as sleeping on the hospital parent's bed night after night was not very comfortable. The gym pass was exactly what was needed on those long chemotherapy days when Sebastian wanted me out of his hair, even though he had no hair. (I could not resist that pun.) Only cancer patients and ex-cancer patients can make cancer jokes like that.

The hospital discounted parking for their long-term patients, but the daily fee was adding up. After many months of long hospital stays, I discovered the **Abbey Solo Foundation**. This foundation was set up in honour of a little girl who had sadly lost her battle with cancer. Her foundation runs regular sausage sizzles in honour of her memory, raising funds to help families pay for hospital parking and other necessities such as food, fuel, travel vouchers and emergency accommodation. I received some parking vouchers to help with these costs. If you visit Bunnings one weekend, look out for the Abbey Solo Foundation. Purchase a sausage and know the money will go to a great cause.

Sebastian mentioned my love of coffee. In the early days of treatment, I spent a small fortune on coffee to get me through the long days. Then, I was kindly given a free coffee card courtesy of **Koala Kids Foundation** to use at the cafe on the ground floor of the hospital. Anyone who loves coffee would know that feeling of joy when they drink that perfect drop. Koala Kids delivered regular meals and groceries to our

The ~~Worst~~ Best Year

home. I was extremely blessed to have my mum and in-laws help with the housework and the preparation of meals but some days we didn't even have time to put a load of washing on. Coming home and finding ready-made meals or basic groceries was a godsend. They also sent Sebastian a smash cake for his birthday, Christmas and Easter hampers, and gingerbread houses.

Starlight Children's Foundation was like the Fairy Godmother of wishes. They worked hard to keep Sebastian's spirits up throughout his entire treatment, bringing joy through their Starlight Express Room, a room in the hospital to entertain young children and their families, as well as through their Wishgranting Program. The Starlight Express Room was limited and not at total capacity when we were there because of COVID restrictions, but the restrictions were beginning to lift towards the end of our visits. It is so lovely to see that the restrictions are now mostly lifted. Starlight TV is a channel that is broadcast throughout the hospital that entertains children from their beds. However, Sebastian always did prefer his Youtube. Sebastian's Starlight Wish was to meet Rafael Nadel and attend the Australian Open. Unfortunately, the meet and greet did not occur as yet again, COVID rules were stringent at best.

He did however receive the most amazing Australian Open experience. Our family was given a couple of nights, all expenses paid, at the Crown Casino. We enjoyed all that the Australian Open had to offer. Sebastian was in his element at the tennis, where he could watch the matches unfold in style. To finish off an already fantastic experience, our whole family went to watch the men's Grand Final. Starlight did not

Natalie - So Many Wonderful Charities

only make Sebastian's Australian Open wish come true, but throughout his treatment they provided great motivation and positive distraction by keeping in touch and sending gifts and cards which put a smile on his face. They even sent thoughtful cards to Elijah thanking him for being an amazing little brother.

Challenge thought of everything and had a permanent presence in the hospital. Even with COVID restrictions, they would always check in on us in person or by phone. The wonderful staff used to drop off games and snacks when we were staying overnight. They checked in to see if we needed cleaning or meal services at home. Challenge also provided parents with weekends away. Their mum and dad retreats are amazing and are just what parents need to re-energise to face the next week ahead. The parent's retreat was a great way to connect with other parents who understood what you are going through. They have ongoing camps and holiday programs offered to the patients and siblings. Their Facebook page included images of some camp experiences that look fun and engaging. Challenge gave our family AFL footy and tennis tickets which we used for enjoyment. They run activities involving siblings, which Elijah took advantage of during the school holidays. Christmas 2022, the year we finished treatment, they treated us to a week away at their beachside property in Blairgowrie on the Mornington Peninsula. It was the perfect week away and just what our family needed to regroup after what we had been through. Challenge has a number of properties located in different locations which have all been gifted to them over the years, all utilised by families for free.

The ~~Worst~~ Best Year

The Blood Bank had a big hand in saving Sebastian's life. Sebastian's treatment would have been significantly delayed without the Blood Bank. Sebastian's haemoglobin levels would have remained dangerously low. Their blood supply is always severely low, but they always manage to save many lives. George has always been a blood donor. I wish that I could be too but as I have had blood cancer, I will sadly never be able to donate. My eldest son Jerome has become a regular donor since Sebastian finished treatment. We do not even have to remind him; he simply books himself in and donates his precious blood.

After finishing treatment, Sebastian wanted to give back, so he joined the *Herald/Sun* Run For The Kids to raise funds for the best hospital in the world. You hear so much about this hospital but cannot understand its brilliance unless you have experienced it firsthand. My three boys make me exceptionally proud every day. We have had some curve balls thrown our way, but George and I have done something right in the parenting department, especially when a young man can see the importance of being proactive and giving back.

So many organisations work exceedingly hard when it comes to fundraising. They use the money raised to do so much good. We live in a fortunate country with organisations like the ones previously mentioned, and we also have one of the best hospitals in the world with first-class doctors and facilities. RCH became our home away from home. I remember staying there when Sebastian was a baby when he had to have his tonsils removed. I have seen how much the hospital has developed over the years. This hospital provided us with many

Natalie - So Many Wonderful Charities

comforts when we needed it most. From doctors to nurses, state-of-the-art facilities and many forms of entertainment. Every corner of this hospital is a blessing, and every cent raised contributes to saving lives. I thank God for many blessings, such as the love of family and friends, for wonderful organisations, hospitals, cancer researchers and doctors. I thank God that my boy is healthy once again.

Chapter 21

It's Never Over

~ *Sebastian* ~

Ring, ring, ring! It wasn't the chemo bell ringing this time, but our doorbell. There was a possibility that we would receive visitors today, but it was not likely. Unknown to me at the time though, Mum had entered a Channel 7 *Sunrise* competition on how she would spend $10,000 at Coles supermarket. Her submission was that she would use the money to celebrate my 16th birthday and the end of my chemo treatment. My dad was the first person to reach the front door and opened it to a cheering crowd, along with shouts of celebration. By the time Elijah, Mum, and I had arrived at the door, the crowd who had gathered at our front door had erupted into an organised chaos. There were massive Channel Seven TV cameras everywhere, along with a camera crew. I could see a big fake cheque (for TV purposes) from Coles that read '$10,000'. I turned to the sounds of the Australian Girls Choir singing a song about my mum and how she "always wins". Indeed, in our family she is well known for winning competitions, but we have never won anything that came close to totalling $10,000 from any one of those competitions she had entered.

I didn't really know what to do at this point. James Tobin started asking us questions about the impact that cancer has had on our family and what it meant to be recognised like this for our hardship. Understandably, Mum was quite emotional as we had recently emerged from a very traumatic experience. It was evident that she was trying very hard to hold back her tears, and I didn't know what to do. So I looked up to see the producer. He was making an air hug with his hands, which prompted me to wrap my arms around her in a hug. I am not the affectionate type, especially with how my OCD can make me really uncomfortable touching other people, but with people from around the entire country watching me before they headed off to work, I needed to act like a normal human and at least seem compassionate. So, in light of the situation, I wrapped my arm around her, almost saying we endured this together. During this heartfelt moment of solidarity, the TV presenters couldn't help having a dig at Jerome. "Jerome, if you're watching, get out of bed!" yelled James Tobin.

Somehow, throughout the chaos of the morning, Jerome had managed to remain in bed. He hadn't even come out to check on the noise, despite the loud sound of the choir out the front. "Jerome's obviously a teenager," said one of the presenters. For someone who didn't even make it on camera, Jerome seemed to have stolen the attention of the show. Just when I thought that I had started to feel comfortable with

The ~~Worst~~ Best Year

the situation in our front yard, which included dozens of Coles workers standing on our front lawn, the girl's choir once again erupted in song with, "Natalie always wins, wins, wins. All she does is win!" Jerome was awake, but his bed probably seemed like an easier choice than coming down to the chaos outside.

***

So what happens now? I slowly started to return to my normal self. A month after ringing the hospital bell, I was no longer constantly getting sick, and my blood counts were pushing what might be called the base of the 'normal' range. I had returned to school, ready for face-to-face learning and to finish the year strong with stellar exam results. After all of this, my family came together as one community to celebrate my recovery. As my 16th birthday was soon approaching, my parents thought it would be a great idea to use the $10,000 in Coles vouchers to mark the end of my treatment with a massive celebration at our house. We would invite our entire family and friends, and the invite list totalled 150 people. As Jerome had Year 12 exams around my actual birthday, the party was going to be delayed a week.

That didn't matter since the cancer organisations couldn't bear to miss the fun of my birthday. We had received a big brown box from Koala Kids wrapped in their branded sticky tape, which was a generous birthday surprise. I ran my finger across the tape, searching for where one layer of tape was stacked up on top of the next so I could peel it off with my fingers. Encased in the box was a chocolate dome and a wooden gavel the length of one of those wooden rulers from primary school. I read the congratulatory message and then proceeded to smash the cake with the gavel, careful not to put a hole in the table in the process. Chocolate, lolly snakes, hundreds and thousands, and other sweets went flying over the table and floor in a complete mess. What better way to celebrate turning 16 than to smash some chocolate into pieces? It was only a small get-together with my closest family on the actual day of my birthday and the smash cake was the perfect inclusion for the day. Koala Kids sent us another smash cake on my 17th birthday, forging a tradition of birthday celebrations post-chemo, where I had the chance to live another whole year thanks to the wonderful efforts of the team who looked after me.

In typical Lebanese fashion, my real party was no small event. The invite list itself required an Excel spreadsheet with all of our family who we had considered inviting as if it was a wedding. Every family member who even expressed the slightest consideration for me over the six months of my sickness received an invite. Families who were previously strangers to us who we hadn't seen in years and had reached out to offer their support were invited. Even families from across the country and around the world travelled to Melbourne to attend the party. I heard the doorbell first thing in the morning when my grandmother came over to help prepare for the party. From the moment the guests started to arrive, I didn't catch a break. The doorbell rang throughout the house; I would open it to see guests arriving, greet them, and take the presents that they had brought with them up to my room. Of course, everyone wanted a photo with me, so I would then have to take one while having a quick chat with them. The chat was of course cut short by the sound of the doorbell ringing again. Then I would repeat again and again for a good half an hour.

"I am so proud of you!" Aunty Monique told me. Throughout chemo, I often considered how I didn't appreciate the magnitude of what I was going through, and it was only every so often that it hit me that I had cancer. Now was one of those times, when everyone was gathered to celebrate its end. I began to gain the perspective that cancer was a part of me and who I was; it was part of my new identity. No longer was I 'forgetting' that I had cancer or failing to realise just how much of my life had changed because I was in survival mode. I could now focus on how cancer recast my life in a new light of hope and strengthened my core values for the better. I will not forget this experience, even if I try, not for a second.

Early on in my treatment, Claira told Mum, Dad, and me about an ongoing study based in Adelaide that was aimed at determining genes that predispose people to different cancers, particularly blood cancers. Despite having family members who have been diagnosed with Hodgkin lymphoma, not the most common of cancers, there is yet to be a gene found to predispose you to Hodgkin lymphoma. This study was a chance to find that gene if it was out there. Our family were perfect candidates given the incidence of the condition amongst my relatives, even if you only took my immediate family. Our job was to have a sample of blood taken at the hospital and have 20 hairs mailed to the university in Adelaide, which would be studied to find common genes amongst Hodgkin patients and their families. Since it had been a couple of months after my last chemo session, the hair on my body had grown back, and they were ready to be plucked. I reached for an envelope and began to pull the hairs like leaves off a tree without the use of tweezers.

Mum looked at me strangely. "Sebastian! You need tweezers to pull them out properly!" "No Mum, look, I have the full hair right here."

I didn't realise why she was so surprised that I could pull my hair out so easily. However, since I had still only recently finished chemo, my hair was not too hard to remove, which made plucking them out with my bare hands an easy task. My hope continued like a shooting star as my cultivated efforts to help future cancer patients would not be futile, and eventually, if I continued supporting the community of cancer sufferers, I could really make a difference for them. Meanwhile, I started to become overwhelmed by a sense of imprisonment in my own feelings. When I rang the bell, I felt as though cancer was over. I felt it again at the parties that ensued, and I felt it as I completed the genetic donation, which we had long planned to do as a family at the end of my treatment. Was I ever going to stop feeling this way? How was I going to stop feeling this way? I had lots of questions for my internal monologue, but no answers.

New Year's Eve that year was to be held at my cousins' house in Sydney. Many of my mum's side of the family drove up there with us from Melbourne to ring in the new year together. The drive from Melbourne

The ~~Worst~~ Best Year

to Sydney is a full day's worth, which makes for a decent road trip with the family, all crammed in the same car. It was an uncomfortable trip. Since I had just obtained my learner driver's licence, I could use the road trip as a chance to increase my hours on the road. What better way to do it than driving on the freeway? I had driven around industrial areas with minimal other cars on the road and at very low speeds. I had only amassed a couple of hours of driving at this point and was not accustomed to driving the high speeds that the freeway had to offer. We were a few hours into the trip when my dad needed a break from driving and offered me a turn on the road. As I wanted all the driving experience that I could get, I instantly agreed and he pulled over. We put up the learner plates in the car and I started to drive.

I was pulling out from a stationary position onto a freeway where the speed limit was 110km/h and I had just learned how to turn the steering wheel, so I was incredibly nervous. We waited as cars passed one at a time until Dad told me it was safe to go, and go I did. I slammed my foot down hard on the accelerator, holding on to the shaking steering wheel with a firm grip, and then proceeded to turn off the indicator, not realising that it had already turned itself off. Thus, I accidentally turned the left indicator on. My heart was now starting to edge up past 100 beats per minute as I nervously considered what the car behind me was thinking (and trust me, I know what 100 beats per minute feels like). Out of panic, I reset it by grabbing the indicator with my whole right hand flicking it hard, while holding the wheel with my left. In doing so, I managed to turn the indicator back to the left. I tried again and turned it to the right not knowing how to lightly tap it. This continued a few times until I eventually got it working, and from there my dad set me to cruise control so I only had to hold the wheel straight.

The problem I had with New Year's Eve was the struggles of OCD. The thing about having OCD is that when you are confronted with an intrusive or uncomfortable thought, you have the urge to calm yourself down with thought or action-based rituals known as compulsions. OCD often doesn't make sense and is illogical in nature. I particularly struggled with OCD on New Year's Eve as I always wanted to end a year 'perfectly' and completing compulsions helped me feel pure and perfect (at least in the short term).

This New Year's Eve was a bit different though. I didn't spend hours doing compulsions, but I did spend the hour in the lead-up to midnight reflecting on the year that I had just gone through. While I was grateful for all the positives that came out of cancer, I could only focus on the negatives. I thought about receiving chemo, having my body changed, my bones dying, my life being shaken up and I thought, *Why me? Why did I have to be the one to go through this? Why was I cursed with bad luck?* No one was controlling my fate, but I felt like it would be easier if someone was because then I could become mad at them for what had happened to me. At the same time, I was conflicted in my emotions. I was overwhelmingly proud of my accomplishments in spite of all the obstacles that were thrown my way and the hurdles I had jumped in my battle to overcome cancer. I'd maintained my academic success and put myself in a strong position to do well throughout my senior

The ~~Worst~~ Best Year

studies. My insides were like a pot of 'feeling stew' and I didn't know what I was feeling when they all mixed together.

"Are you good?" my father asked. I shrugged him off and I told him I was fine, I just needed to be alone. My mum then came and tried to talk to me, followed by some uncles and aunties. I wanted to be free from the complex emotions I was experiencing, and talking to them was not helping. I distanced myself from everyone so I could continue to reflect upon the year that I had, alone. Again, I felt a sense of déjà vu as I knew that this year had marked the end of my cancer journey. The countdown to midnight was fast approaching and people were preparing for the countdown. As a group, we worked our way from thirty seconds to zero before we welcomed in 2023. I didn't hug anyone or wish them a happy new year; instead, I ran up the stairs in exaltation as the emotional burden that I was carrying was lifted off my chest and shoulders. I ran outside on the balcony, out into the pouring rain. The thing was that no amount of bucketing droplets of rain was going to overcome my feeling of liberation; I was finally free. The song soon changed to *C'est la Vie*, my favourite song at the time, a fitting way to bring in the new year.

I was moving forward into a post-chemo life where I could celebrate living at every corner I turned. I would attend parties, enjoy my time with family and friends, put in the effort to achieve success, and face a few curveballs along the way. One curveball I wasn't expecting was how slowly some people were to catch up with the new me. Nearly a year on from the end of chemo, people were still congratulating me on completing treatment. 15 months on, and I was talking to some old friends who still didn't know that I had finished treatment. People who hadn't seen me in a while and may not have known I had finished treatment were still running around for me after 18 months.

Today, people's eyes, the same compassionate eyes that once made me feel special, now confuse me. The look they give says they still see me as the cancer kid. It fills me with an uneasy nostalgia, bringing me back to a time that was far from emotionally simple. The first time someone saw me after chemo, they would always act the same way. Maybe they didn't know whether I was still sick and thus weren't sure how to act around me, or maybe they simply wanted to show that they were aware of what I had been through. These individuals would walk on their tippy-toes around me like the floor was a thin layer of ice. They would be extra nice, and offer to get me my food without me having to get up. They never had ill intent, yet their actions somehow were demoralising, almost seeming patronising as they reminded me that I am still the Mr Cancer to them. And suddenly, like I had zapped my cancer out of their memory, the next time they saw me I was once again Sebastian. It's as if they had a mental snapshot of sick Sebastian and it is not until they saw me again after treatment that they updated their mental image of me. When I was sick, people treating me special was the norm, anything less would stand out to me like that one grade I was never proud of. After treatment, as I see the people I haven't seen in years for the first time, their special treatment of me is now the memorable exception.

The ~~Worst~~ Best Year

When I first noticed this after chemo I was guilt-ridden, thinking that I didn't deserve people's sympathy anymore; now I find it amusing that almost two years after I rang that bell, people who are seeing me for the first time still can't shake the thought of Cancer Seb. Ringing the bell was the first and last part of a journey to recovery. What follows me around long after the cancer cells stop dividing is being branded as the Cancer Kid. It is a big white label which everyone can see from miles away. I will forever have my scars where the port once sat in my chest, and the memories formed in the depths of the RCH are now etched into my brain, experiences to remember for many years to come.

My 16th birthday had been a symbolic day that celebrated the end of my treatment and was a chance to move forward. Although I had already celebrated the end of treatment when I rang the bell, and then when people came to see me that night and in the coming days, it had been a way to say a final goodbye to cancer, surrounded by many people who supported me on my journey. But I found myself trying to make sense of what exactly marked the end of treatment. Was it the 16th birthday party? Or maybe the blood and hair donations that we provided to the cancer study; my follow-up scans; the end of the year celebrations in Sydney; 6 months after treatment when I had my vaccines due to my lost immunity from treatment; when I had my wisdom teeth removed the following year which was put off because of my treatment; or was it when I had recovered from the health deficits from chemo and had the port used to administer it removed?

Thinking about all of these events, I came to realise that I didn't want the journey with cancer to be over and that it never really is. I like to be a stand-out, unique person. I have been permanently transformed in so many ways, mentally, physically, and spiritually from my cancer experiences, altering the course of my life. The scars where my port was removed are there as are my memories of 2022, but maybe these aren't so bad. I am now left with the long-lasting effects of chemo on my body, the wisdom learned in the hospital about the precious nature of life, and the sense of purpose I now have to help people who are as ill as I once was. I now feel a calling to bolster blood drives at my school, and support initiatives that improve life for cancer patients. The journey of cancer started when I was itching my guts out, but it doesn't finish when the chemo stops—it continues as long as I keep it alive. Perhaps a life as an oncologist awaits me.

Chapter 22

Finding A New Normal

~ *Natalie* ~

    To see these words formed on paper is a testament to the persistence and determination of the human spirit. This is a tangible representation of our thoughts, feelings and experiences, and achieving this through words carries a profound sense of accomplishment. We wrote this in the face of adversity so that you could understand what we went through as individuals and as a family. It is not just a story; it was our designated path that documented our struggles and trials, but ultimately, we found the strength to overcome all the obstacles we faced.

    It wasn't until we were well into writing this story that I finally found the courage to read what Sebastian had written. Initially, I avoided reading his part as I thought knowing how he felt would have made me too sad, and I was not ready to experience this. I also didn't want his writing or his recollection of events to influence mine. I was proud of how he expressed himself through words. What stood out for me was that I noticed that he referred to his cancer experience as a journey. Although he experienced sickness, pain and fear, he looked at it through the eyes of learning and building his knowledge and curiosity. In contrast, I viewed our experiences as an obstacle, one we should never have endured. Although we lived under the same roof and travelled on a similar road, we viewed our experiences very differently.

When we are faced with tragedy in our lives we never really return to normal. We learn to create a new normal. Life never goes back to the way it was. I felt that way after my cancer diagnosis. Even though treatment had finished for me, I did not experience the feeling of normality until many months had passed and maybe not even until years later. Just like Sebastian felt on New Years Eve the year he finished treatment, I too had a similar experience. I remember New Year's Eve 2014. We had just counted down to midnight and a wave of emotions overcame me. I remember thinking, what will 2015 bring? Will I be cancer-free? The fear of my cancer returning consumed my thoughts, but I was not going to let these thoughts drown me. Slowly, you begin to adjust to your new normal and when you start to feel slight improvements, life takes you on yet another turn.

For me, it was my father passing away. This was the second time I had experienced that white noise I spoke about earlier. When Dad passed away, I recall dropping in a heap to the floor of the foyer of the hospital. I was a complete mess. People were speaking to me and trying to console me, but I did not register their words. This hit me harder than my cancer diagnosis. I had a very special bond with my dad. He was my superhero, and he left me without warning. I felt a real void in my life. The night before his heart attack, I was at his house celebrating my mum and nephew's combined birthdays. My dad was so happy and full of life. It happened so quickly and without warning. One month earlier, my father, a man who was bigger than life, was dancing and singing with me at my 40th birthday party, then a month later, he was gone. This was something I really struggled to come to terms with. I felt so sad for so long. Watching my mother's grief was heartbreaking and I knew that life would never be the same again. I had my family distract me and with time, I found strength and learned yet again to find a new normal.

Then, that horrible day in March 2022 broke my spirits. My son was diagnosed with cancer. This time, I never believed I could return to a new normal from this earth-shattering revelation. At 15, he should have been hanging out with his friends and not bound to a hospital bed. I cried many tears, but there were times we laughed so hard it hurt. We bonded during this time as many hours were spent together watching Wimbledon in the middle of the night or playing *Bananagrams*. I rarely beat him when we played that game. At that time, finding a new normal was really hard. While Sebastian was going through treatment, I was rolling with the punches, and there were many punches. I admit in the early days of diagnosis I struggled emotionally, but I pulled myself together to be a mother to him during one of the most challenging times of our lives. I spoke to a counsellor at the hospital, and it helped. I also received some private counselling sessions via Zoom. I had to be strong for him to be his support person. I had no energy to give to my other two boys or my husband because my only focus was getting Sebastian well again. I knew that they understood.

Once Sebastian had finished treatment, I struggled to find that new normal again. I had mother's guilt. I blamed myself that I may have carried the gene that I had passed on to my child. I experienced the guilt of not identifying the signs of Sebastian's cancer sooner. I deeply regret not being there for my other two boys. Jerome was completing Year 12 at the time, the most important year of his school life, and I was not there for him. Instead, he was there for me. Jerome ensured he was home for his younger brother Elijah and helped me with tasks around the house. Jerome had just turned 18 and wanted to go out with friends. Yet, I put so much unnecessary pressure on Jerome every time he went out to be careful where he went and who he went with as Sebastian was so immunocompromised and there was always the fear of COVID coming home. My behaviour was so unfair to him, but he never complained.

There were many nights when Sebastian's temperature peaked, and his heart was racing. I was stressed taking his observations and speaking to the fast-track cancer ward on the phone. Jerome was always by my side, willing to lend a helping hand or just be there to offer his support. Elijah, who was only 11 years old at the time, needed his mother. I was not there for him either. I missed school assemblies and couldn't take him to birthday parties and after-school activities. I am so blessed that my boys understood and never complained. They both knew the seriousness of the situation, and they just rolled with it. Getting back to a new normal after all this guilt was challenging.

I felt guilty for being frustrated and for taking out these angry emotions on my husband, George, who bore it all. Sebastian would take his frustrations out on me and I would do the same to George. People get married for many reasons. I say marry your best friend. This may sound really cliché, but it is true. You can marry someone handsome and rich who makes you laugh, but if tragedy strikes, all the money in the world won't save you. I married my best friend, and once the storm passed, we could sail the calm sea together. Obviously, I thought George was very hot when we started dating (I needed to add this line because he will read this). I agree that there needs to be an initial attraction. We had been friends for so long before anything else, and we spoke for long hours on the phone. We built a strong foundation before marriage and children. When life threw us curve balls, there was no one else I wanted by my side except for George. If we married solely for passion, that would have dissipated when I was receiving treatment and couldn't even look at myself in the mirror. While Sebastian was undergoing treatment, our friendship was more important than ever. When we found time to be together, I was either crying, sleeping, taking my emotions out on him or just not talking. Affection was non-existent, yet we fell more in love with each other during the most challenging times of our lives, which is a testament to the strength of our relationship. Marriages can fall apart during adversity. We became stronger together. I never felt tested in our marriage and never questioned our relationship. I felt our love grow through each obstacle that we faced. I was loved, cherished, supported and respected.

Even with George's support, getting back to a new normal after Sebastian's diagnosis was difficult. I required professional help. The counselling in those early days helped me with techniques to calm my mind and regulate my breathing. It helped me to be open and honest about my fears with someone I did not know. Once Sebastian's chemotherapy finished, I thought that I could stop the sessions but a couple of months after his treatment ended, I would still cry with no real cause for my tears. I would become easily angered and avoid people who complained about trivial things. I would snap at shop assistants if I felt they were not doing their jobs properly. I felt like I was losing myself. I had to decide whether I needed to return to therapy.

I sorted through the information I received from the RCH and found a brochure from Redkite. They offered a family counselling program called Cascade, where you met up with other parents once a week and participated in a 90-minute session on dealing with your trauma. This program helped as I was able to express my feelings in a safe environment amongst others who had shared a similar trauma to me. I learned techniques that helped me to move forward. I do not know if I have entirely found my new normal, but I know that I am improving every day. There is only so much one person can handle, and I needed professional help to find myself again. There is no shame in that at all. Life is hard, and it does not matter how strong a person is; sometimes, we just need help.

The ~~Worst~~ Best Year

We are still attending numerous appointments, as Sebastian has had gum and teeth issues after treatment. He has had so many specialist dental appointments. There have been many follow-up oncology appointments, and Sebastian has started to see an orthopaedic specialist who looks after the AVN in his bones. Every time Sebastian looks tired, I become stressed. When he scratches his head because he may have dandruff, I look over to see if he continues to scratch. Every time Sebastian scratches, a knot of anxiety forms in my stomach. He is a naturally early sleeper, but I become worried if he heads off to bed extra early. Every time he feels pain, I worry that it is the AVN in his bones that has developed. When we take him for routine scans, I panic when the phone rings as we await his results. Could it be Mum calling to say hello, or is the hospital calling to inform us of bad news? This is my new normal, but I have come to accept it. My son is cancer-free, thank God, and I need to keep these fears at bay. If this is my new normal, I will learn to live with it as long as my family is happy and healthy.

Simply Put

~ Sebastian ~

Being diagnosed with Hodgkin lymphoma was the most physically and one of the most mentally challenging experiences I have endured. Whilst I had unending confidence in the medical team looking after me and rarely entertained the thought of death, my journey through cancer was not free from burden. Going through chemotherapy often involved spending days on end, unable to decide whether I would rather be as nauseous as I was on one day or experience the torturous agony that paralysed my body on the next. I endured the suffering of chemo-induced AVN, where the bones in my pelvis, femur, tibia, and other lower body regions began to die. Moreover, forced to reconcile with the inevitable isolation associated with undergoing chemotherapy, I found myself in a state of constant mental affliction. In the few instances of reprieve from my isolation when I was able to break free from my online learning routine to attend school, I was frequently condemned to a hospital bed in

The ~~Worst~~ Best Year

the days that ensued as I became deeply sick. Illness was a constant and I was sometimes even forced to overcome multiple pathogens at once.

The chemotherapy essential to my recovery also left my family in an everlasting state of worry. They were worried about my recovery, they were worried about my mental well-being, worried about what would happen when my bone marrow eventually failed to do its job and I would require a blood transfusion. Above all, I was worried about all that I had missed out on during my recovery, and not performing at my best. Cancer gets all the attention as it defines so many people, but it is only a small part of one's life and struggles. I didn't choose to have cancer, but I sure made the most of the journey. Not a single part of me didn't suffer during my six months of chemotherapy, but the experiences I gained would prove to be invaluable parts of my life. Most people see the devil in cancer, but they fail to see the full extent of its impact. Cancer is a wake-up call, it unites families, it pushes you to do things you have never done before, it blesses you with memories that can last a lifetime, it gives you a sense of purpose and most importantly, cancer reminds you of who and what is most important in your life. Ultimately, some might say that I was unlucky to be diagnosed with cancer at the age of 15, but to them I respond that I couldn't be luckier, as it was the greatest experience of my life. This truly was *the best year*!

To continue following our story, please head over to our Instagram page. Our goal is to continue to raise awareness for a cause we are passionate about and help others find the support they need.

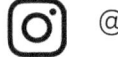 @theworstbestyear

www.ingramcontent.com/pod-product-compliance
Lightning Source LLC
Chambersburg PA
CBHW062046290426
44109CB00027B/2745